Acne Free in 3 Days™

How I Cured My Acne Condition in 3 Days

By Chris Gibson

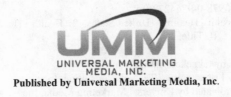

UNIVERSAL MARKETING MEDIA, INC.

Published by Universal Marketing Media, Inc.

Acne Free in 3 Days™

How I Cured My Acne Condition In 3 Days

By Chris Gibson

Published By Universal Marketing Media, Inc. in association with Chris Gibson.

 Universal Marketing Media, Inc. is a publishing and marketing company. 1216 Raymilton Rd., Polk, PA 16342, U.S.A.

The Universal Marketing Media logo is a trademark of Universal Marketing Media, Inc. Visit our website at http://www.universalmarketingmedia.com. Printed in the United States of America

Chris Gibson
http://www.acnefreein3days.com
chrisg@acnefreein3days.com

Gibson, Chris
        Acne free in 3 days™ / How I cured my acne condition in 3 days / Chris Gibson.
                p.   cm.
                Includes bibliographical references and index.
                ISBN 978-0-9764272-0-9
                1. Health - Healing – United States. 2. Health - Healing – Canada.
I. Gibson, Chris. II. Title.

Website design by teknekconsulting.com.
Book design by Fritz Conroy / TekNek Consulting, Inc
Production coordinated by Universal Marketing Media, Inc

Dedication

This book is dedicated to acne sufferers from all around the globe. Most of all it's dedicated to you, our reader— the acne free customer of tomorrow.

Acknowledgements

Thanks to our many clients for the contributions they have made to this work. Without their thirst for information and their faith, I wouldn't have been challenged to dig so deeply, to probe so many crannies, and to look beyond the readily available answers for a true natural solution.

To the entire staff of Universal Marketing Media, Inc., I say a hearty, "Thank you." You are a unique group of caring and competent people. Thanks for being who and what you are. Without you guys, I could never have completed this on time.

Additionally, I wish to acknowledge the countless individuals, organizations, and companies who so generously gave of their time and ideas. **Acne Free in 3 Days**[TM]: *How I Cured My Acne Condition in 3 Days* not only grew from my own experiences, but also from the experiences of many others. Sincerest thanks to everyone!

About the Author

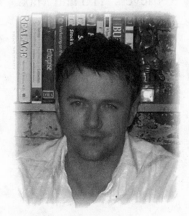

Over the years, Chris Gibson has been able to write several books on alternative healthcare. When Chris first began his career as an author, his first book was about a completely different subject, advertising. However, the huge success of the advertising book led him to take advantage of the opportunity to share his knowledge of effective "all-natural, drugless therapies."

For many years, Chris battled with his acne problems, enduring countless visits to his doctors, drug therapies, and over-the-counter products. These standard methods didn't work for Chris and do not work for a large portion of the population. After much research and fruitless attempts, Chris finally happened on a method that not only clears acne in just days, regardless of how long you have had it, but also does it without the use of drugs or harsh creams.

The all-natural methods described in Chris' book attacks the acne at its source, not just the symptoms. You will be truly amazed by the results you will see just as thousands of his customers, including celebrities and dignitaries, have.

Chris lives on his ranch near Pittsburgh, Pennsylvania, where he spends his non-writing time in his organic gardens, traveling, and training his two Labrador Retrievers, Tiki and Max.

Other Titles Published by Universal Marketing Media

Anyone who has ever been awakened by his or her partner while sleeping or woke up in the morning feeling like they did not get a good nights rest, understands snoring is a serious problem. Although there are literally hundreds of different snoring aids, devices, and pills available on the market, thousands of people still suffer from snoring each year. Juan Walker was also one of these people until he decided to try a different approach. In the book, ***Stop Your Snoring Now™: How I Naturally Cured My Snoring Condition for Life***, Juan shows you how he easily stopped snoring permanently and how you can do the same. Get your own copy today by clicking on the link below.

http://www.stopyoursnoringnow.com

No More Moles, Warts, or Skin Tags™: How I Safely Removed Moles, Warts, and Skin Tags for Life. Best selling holistic author, Chris Gibson, shows you how to remove your moles, warts and skin tags painlessly and easily, with a proven, all-natural method in as little as three days. This method does not require the use of expensive surgeries or useless over-the-counter products. With an almost 100% rate of success, you, too, can be mole, wart and skin tag free for life. Click below to read more about this book and to get your own copy today!

http://www.molewartremoval.com

With over five hip surgeries, numerous complications, and the early onset of osteoarthritis, Nancy MacGranahan knows what the pain of arthritis is all about. In her book, *Arthritis Free for Life™*, Nancy shares her story of how she ended the pain in one month naturally and provides you with the fountain of relief that even has some doctors in the medical profession completely amazed. This does not involve a change in diet, exercise routines, or impossible regimens to follow. This method has worked for the thousands of clients who have read Nancy's book, and it will work for you, too. Click on the link below to read more about this book!

http://www.arthritisfreeforlife.com

Rapid Weight Loss by the Numbers™. Everyone knows being overweight is the number one crippler of health in America today. Although increasing numbers of Americans are overweight, it does not have to be this way. This effective and thoughtful plan for weight loss provides results for individuals of all ages. The author, Chris Gibson, shares with you how he was able to lose 28 pounds and three pants sizes in only three weeks, and how you can do the same without using any worthless diet plans, pills, or supplements. A must read for anyone struggling to lose the weight and keep it off permanently. Get your own copy today!

http://www.weightlossbythenumbers.com

Cold Sore Freedom in 3 Days™: How I Permanently and Safely Cured My Cold Sores for Life. Anyone who has suffered with cold sores knows how embarrassing and frustrating, let alone painful, they can be. The author, Grace Melgarejo, knows your pain because she dealt with cold sores for over 12 years. In her book, she shares her painful story and shows you how you can easily cure your cold sores or herpes simplex I virus in only three days, by using an all-natural method. This method has worked for the thousands of clients who have read Grace's book, and it will work for you, too! Get your own copy today by clicking on the link below.

http://www.coldsorefreedomin3days.com

How I Banished My Bad Breath and Gum Disease for Life. If you are one of the millions of people who struggle with mouth, gum or breath problems, then this is the book for you. The methods outlined in this book do what sprays, mints, and mouth washes cannot do. Included is a widely available but little known cure for even the most pervasive oral health issues. The methods will help you to banish your bad breath and gum disease permanently. The results are scientifically proven, easy and pleasant to attain and 100% effective. Click on the link below to read more about this book and to get your own copy today!

http://www.banishbadbreath.com

Table of Contents

How I Finally Cleared My Adult Acne

My name is Chris Gibson. I am a business professional with a very successful business and very active personal life and the author of several books. I have owned my own businesses as well as served in the role of vice president in several companies. I've dealt with the CEOs and boards of companies—presenting their services in high profile situations. I have spent time in the public eye.

For me - My APPEARANCE IS EVERYTHING!

Physical appearance is actually important for just about everyone, a fact that research in the social sciences is only now beginning to show us. We are often judged by the way we look. That crucial first impression is very real and is important in business, entertainment, employment, and social situations.

For whatever reason (and there are a lot of theories about this), people tend to respond more favorably to attractive people than they do to people perceived as less attractive. Social scientists even have a name for this response: the "halo effect." According to Dr. Mona Phillips, who teaches sociology at Spellman College, the "halo effect" refers to the tendency to associate a cluster of positive characteristics with a positive physical appearance. "People assume that if someone is attractive, then they have [other] good qualities [as well]" (Phillips 2001).

I believe the opposite effect is also true, too; people who are seen as less than attractive often face subtle discrimination and are unconsciously judged as less intelligent, less clean, less trustworthy, and less capable than others. Like it or not, "we live in a culture that places a high premium on external appearances" ("Do Attractive People" 2001).

Some sociologists believe that attractiveness may have an evolutionary explanation that has to do with "the link between beauty and health. . . . Attractiveness is preferred because it is associated with health" (Moghaddam 2003). On the other hand, anything that suggests illness or imperfection, blemishes or scars, is, often unconsciously, not tolerated by the "tribe" we live in.

One of the most common problems associated with appearance—and yet one of the most devastating—is acne. In American alone, "[a]n estimated 17 to 28 million people have some degree of acne; 7 million have at least moderately intense activity, and 750,000 have more severe inflammation" (Stern 1992).

As early as 1948, dermatologists recognized the seriousness of this often casually dismissed problem: "There is no single disease which causes more psychic trauma . . . more general feeling of inferiority and greater sums of psychic suffering than does *acne vulgaris* [common acne]" (Sultzberger and Zaidens 1948). In fact, the social acceptance of people with acne is getting much worse. According to Dr. Richard G. Fried, a noted dermatologist, "There is no tolerance whatsoever for imperfection [today]. Blemishes are more difficult than ever to live with."

Even so, not until very recently, have acne and the acne sufferer been given the kind of attention they deserve. "The reasons for this [lack of attention] are many. After all, everyone gets acne to one degree or another . . . In most cases, it goes away on its own. While it is running its course, it is not a serious threat to anyone's overall health" (American Academy of Dermatology 2005). Even so, for the acne sufferer, the affliction can leave serious and sometimes permanent physical, emotional, and psychological scars.

What I am about to share with you is my own personal experience with what I can only call my "battle" with acne. Like many people, I spent agonizing years and thousands of dollars trying just about everything.

Dermatologists are expensive. Among the most expensive of all M.D.s, they have an average annual income of around $290,000. Furthermore, because skin care has become such a big business, the normal "wait time to see a dermatologist in major cities around the country is 24.3 days—the longest among [the] high-demand medical specialties including obstetrics and gynecology and cardiology" (Merritt).

Antibiotics—which commonly cause nausea—and other prescription medication is also costly (Acutane/isitretinoin, for example, can cost a staggering $450 for one-hundred pills). Moreover, prescribed medications involve months of treatment, give only limited relief, and often have dangerous side effects (Acutane/isitretinoin, one particularly dangerous though popular drug, will be discussed in detail later).

While hundreds of over-the-counter products are available, few provide any lasting effects, even though the cosmetic industry makes millions of dollars yearly selling their promised cures and flawless complexions. We have all seen the air-brushed magazine pictures of both female and male models, with captions claiming miraculous cures with this or that facial cream, astringent, or moisturizer.

Unfortunately, these claims prove ineffective in all but the mildest cases of acne. Sufferers of moderate to severe acne, after months, even years, of expensive treatment, usually find themselves back where they started from. Remarkably, I finally was able to cure my serious acne problem on my own with a natural program that took only three days to complete.

You may be thinking, "If that's true Chris, then why doesn't everyone know about this?" Well, the answer is simple.

Many people DO know about this in certain circles, but unfortunately, as you may already know, many effective alternative therapies that work are shunned until they become so popular that science has to research, prove, and then recognize their worth.

Only in recent years, for instance, has the ancient Chinese therapy of acupuncture been accepted by the medical community in the United States.

"The National Institute of Health Consensus Conference (November 5, 1997) concluded that clear evidence supports the efficacy of acupuncture in the control of chemotherapy-related nausea . . . ."

Medical research, especially in the United States, is notoriously conservative and reluctant to accept new approaches. Like many alternatives to standard chemical-based medicines and practice, information and discoveries in alternative healthcare and holistic medicine are usually not widely shared.

Nonetheless, alternative approaches to disease and health have been used successfully for centuries. Scientists have discovered that people in different countries have used similar herbs and plants for healing, suggesting that these remedies are readily available and effective.

Alternative healthcare (sometimes referred to as "holistic healthcare") is based on a philosophy that looks at the whole person and the relationship between the parts of the body and the whole body. General medicine and pharmacology have traditionally focused on the individual part, the diseased or injured area of the body and the individual ailment. Alternative healthcare—as you will see from my experience—takes a different approach, believing that the part never functions alone.

What happens to one organ or area of the body involves the whole body, and how the whole body functions is a reflection of the individual parts working in health and harmony. Likewise, ailments—and their cures—affect the whole organism.

21

Holistic approaches to healing and good health are accepted in many advanced countries, especially in Europe, and, to a lesser extent, in the United States. "In Germany, some 600 to 700 plant-based medicines are available and are prescribed by approximately 70 percent of German physicians" ("Herbal Medicine" 2002). The popularity in the United States in recent years of St. John's wart (*Hypericum perforatum*) for the treatment of mild depression and of Echinacea (*Echinacea pururea*) to boost the immune system and to relieve flu-like symptoms offer proof that alternative approaches do find their way into our healthcare system.

You probably read about this all the time. In fact, up until 20 years ago, few doctors of any specialty even recommended a person take simple multi-vitamins. Now days, they "see" the benefit and have changed course. This happens all the time.

What I am sharing with you actually *has* been **verified** many times and **written** about extensively by such doctors as Dr. Harold J. Reily and William A. McGarey M.D., just to name a few. (Dr. McGarey has written extensively on the work of Dr. Edgar Cayce who is considered the founder of the holistic healthcare movement in America.) Alternative medicine has also been recognized by the National Institutes of Health (NIH), which set up the Office of Alternative Medicine (OAM) in 1992. The OAM spends $3 million a year "exploring unconventional healing techniques such as meditation, massage, vitamin therapy and herbal therapy" (holisticoline.com).

The willingness to consider alternative approaches has even received some minimal acceptance by health insurers, including a pilot program at Mutual of Omaha and a Blue Cross of Washington policy that covers naturopathy and homeopathy (holisticonline.com).

Some doctors in the medical profession are willing to look beyond the symptoms. They are willing to acknowledge there are many alternative therapies out there that can heal—often without the serious side effects that drugs, as we shall see, bring with them. In fact, 70 percent of primary care physicians indicate they would like some training in complementary and alternative medicine (Berman 1995), and 80 percent of medical students would like to have such training (Jonas 1997).

Patients themselves have taken the initiative to seek out alternative therapies and medicine. In 1990, according to the New England Journal of Medicine, one in three patients in America used some form of alternative therapy. The number of visits to alternative health care practitioners that year was 425 million, more than the number of visits made to biomedical (traditional) doctors that year. Clearly, more and more patients are willing to try alternative approaches to healing and health maintenance.

You probably know that acne is a ***tough*** disease to cure through traditional biomedical approaches, or you would not still be searching for an answer—I was the same way. The road for me personally to conquer it finally was a long and very personal experience.

Who gets acne? Well, just about 100 percent of the population between 12 and 17 gets some acne. (Even King Tut, the "boy king" who ruled Egypt in 1355 B.C. and who died at 17, had it—jars of Egyptian herbal pimple remedies were found in his tomb!)

The word "acne" itself is a distortion of the ancient Greek word "acme," which means "point" or "peak." Adolescence—the time of life during which acne becomes a problem—was considered by the ancient Greeks to be the "peak" of one's life.

In most cases, "acne appears as an occasional white head or black head or pimple. It doesn't seem to prefer one race or ethnic group to another; females and males are affected about equally—males are maybe slightly more likely to get it. The only accurate predictor of acne and its severity seems to be family history (Levine 2005).

Outbreaks can be expected for about five years after the acne first makes its appearance. For most people, it is no longer a problem after the early 20s. For some reason, though, dermatologists are seeing more and more patients with severe acne into their late 20s and 30s.

According to one dermatologist, "We are seeing an epidemic of adult acne, so the old rules that 'just hang in till you're 18 or 20 and you'll outgrow your acne' are absolutely gone. I have more 35-year-old women in my practice than teenagers" (Fried).

Even though everyone experiences acne at one time or another, the invisible effects of acne are rarely discussed.

A recent poll conducted by the American Counseling Association (ACS) showed that only about 28 percent of teenage girls are willing to discuss the problem even with their mothers (Levine). The shame and guilt associated with severe acne is best summed up in the words of Chelsea Fahey, a former Miss Teen America: "I was so ashamed. It was like if I talked about it, I was admitting that it was there, and I didn't want to do that" (Levine).

I share my story today because many people say they recognize themselves in my experiences and are able to gain insight and, more important, relief from it. They are no longer alone in their battle with acne.

I try to look at my experience with acne as a journey. My goal is to help you become acne free just as I have been able to do. I have written extensively on all kinds of maladies that befall us as human beings.

I have written on alternatives that work for such things as losing weight, clearing other skin conditions naturally, and co-authored several more books. (I have included a list of my best selling books and others we publish at the beginning for you.)

As you can see, I have had my share of issues even though the medical community would call me very healthy by their tests and standards. I do not have any major health issues, thank goodness, and have been blessed with strength and superb health in the major areas.

However, like everyone else, I have had a few battles. My books, and those my company publishes, are designed to address many of these conditions. I am grateful for being able to have the gift of sharing.

To me, it is the so-called "chronic conditions" such as being overweight, migraines, skin conditions and so on, which are what affect our quality of life the most. They may not "kill" us, but they certainly take away from the life we were meant to enjoy.

This book on clearing acne naturally is wildly popular because it educates and helps from the level of experience of having "lived" it. The methods work, and they work by allowing you to take charge of your own health solution. There is, of course, a little work you have to do and some directions to follow—a small price to pay.

Everything always has a price, and it rarely has to do with money. I talk to thousands of people each month on various issues like acne, and it always fascinates me how our feelings about it are always the same.

Yet, someone always is not willing to ***pay the price,*** no matter how easy. I get asked all the time how is it possible that my complexion is so clear and young looking (I am 40 now).

For example, let's say that you want to have a complexion and body like Brad Pitt (if you're a guy) or Cindy Crawford (if you are a lady). You're going to have to *work out* a little; you're going to have to spend some time lifting weights, and you are going to have to watch what you eat.

You just might have to change some things that you are doing now. You can't eat pizza everyday or drink a case of beer and expect no effects. You are going to have to take responsibility for your choices and then the improvements will be seen.

An old but useful saying (attributed to just about everyone from Ben Franklin to Gandhi) tells us that "we dig our graves with our teeth." Certainly this proverb is nowhere more true than in America in the twenty-first century. According to Michael McGinnis, M.D., of the Robert Wood Johnson Foundation, our unhealthy dietary habits are built into the American way of life, and "systematically, over the last 50 years, we have engineered physical activity out of our environment."

Food—especially junk food—is everywhere. Junk foods, as most of us know by now, are simply those foods that have little if any nutritional value, foods that have "empty calories." These foods are usually high in sugar, salt, and/or fat content.

As astonishing as it may sound, "40 percent of Americans' daily diet [consists] of sugar, fats and oils. . . " (Clapp 2005).

The average American eats about 120 pounds of sugar a year (that's about the weight of a petite, 5'3," twenty-five-year-old woman). Is it any wonder that 60 million adult Americans are obese? Worse, 14% of all adolescents and 13% of all children are overweight or obese ("Journey to Wellness").

In addition to their bad food habits, Americans are becoming more and more sedentary and lazy. (Unfortunately, the "couch potato" is not just a funny stereotype anymore. It describes too many Americans, both young and old.) According to Ruth Kava, Director of Nutrition at the American Council on Science and Health, some of the most significant changes in the activity levels of American have come about since the computer revolution—especially since the introduction of the Internet.

Instead of going to the library to get information, we can now "Google" our way to almost anything we want to know about. And children now spend hours on computer games and computer-related schoolwork; hours that in many cases used to be spent outside playing. . . .Many do not have regular gym classes in school any more.

On the home front, we have remote control for our televisions so we don't have to move to change channel or volume. Our appliances are ever more labor-saving and lighter. Even cars are easier to drive than . . . in the days before automatic transmissions, power steering, power brakes, and power seats, drivers had to use a few more calories to parallel park, adjust seat position, and just drive. Although these changes are each small in and of themselves, they add up over time—and so do the calories they save. (2005)

Clearly, changes in our lifestyles have created serious health issues overall. Some especially pessimistic observers even believe that "today's children are on their way to becoming the first generation in modern times who will have a shorter life expectancy than their parents" (Clapp 2005). As another observer puts it, "Perhaps more powerfully than any other single factor, our daily food choices determine whether [we] are basically healthy, vital and strong or . . .suffer with average health and eventually fall victim to illness and disease."

The same may be true for your acne condition. If certain foods aggravate your acne condition, you might have to stop eating them. That is called "paying the price."

Could you pay it for a clear and youthful complexion? Could you pay it to feel better about yourself?

Listen to this comment from a young woman with acne:

I don't look in mirrors. . . I am like a vampire—I shy away from mirrors. I comb my hair using my silhouette on the wall to show the outline of my head. I have not looked myself in the eyes in years, and [it] is painful not to be able to do that, and that is a direct result of acne, the acne scarring. (Patient testimony courtesy of John Koo, M.D., cited in "The Social Impact of Acne")

Would you pay it to look in the mirror and smile back at yourself?

I have a very good friend in Dallas who is a very nice guy and highly intelligent. He is 38. When I come down and we go out, he gets very annoyed as I get my ID checked over and over. He's also annoyed when all the women talk to me instead of him.

He is overweight, about 30 pounds, and does nothing to take care of his skin. He still breaks out with pimples and has eczema. Don't get me wrong, he has great hygiene, but he doesn't work out or exercise, and he eats a lot of junk.

It's not easy, and it is getting harder to make good choices. Americans are eating out more and exercising less than ever before. For a while, the fast food industry seemed to be helping people by providing good—or at least improved—food choices on their menus.

The better-for-you food pendulum that so quickly changed the look of fast-food menus and that's often credited with changing consumer eating habits nationwide appears to be swinging back. Or maybe it never really swung away from indulgence in the first place. (Horovitz)

Worse still, in recent months, the fast food industry actually seems to be challenging the healthy lifestyle. One fast food chain has come out with—and even flaunts—its new burger that has 1,420 calorie and enough fat grams for the average person for a whole week!

The fast food industry defends its position by pointing out that the healthy items they have added to the menu have sold very poorly.

According to one fast food CEO, "These [unhealthy] products sell better than health-conscious products. We don't tell consumers what they want. They tell us" (Horovitz).

My friend, like a lot of Americans, simply does not pay attention to the longstanding advice that the choices he makes about exercise and diet are important. In fact, over the last decade, the picture has gotten worse for most of us. Similar studies done in 1990 and 1999 show that "the [negative] impact of poor diet and lack of physical activity has increased [over the decade]" (Wood 2004).

I believe that most of us are not aware of the seriousness and the extensiveness of our bad habit, how our unhealthy lifestyles affect our whole society. Ken Clapp, CEO of Medical Mutual of Ohio, recently wrote an article for *The Columbus Dispatch*, in which he discussed the cost of Americans' bad habits. Mr. Clapp argued that health insurance companies cannot possibly absorb the cost of illnesses and injuries that result from the growing trend of Americans to ignore the benefits of a healthy lifestyle— the cost, he implies will have to be borne by all of us.

[W]e exercise too little, we eat too much, and on top of it all, many of us continue to smoke even though we all know the devastating effect smoking has on health and health-care costs (Clapp).

It is estimated that the actual cost of smoking, taking into consideration disabilities and treatment that result from smoking, is about $40 per pack of cigarettes smoked! (Incidentally, every pack costs the smoker about two hours of his or her life!)

Mr. Clapp continues: "we must learn to associate the cost of health care with the way we choose to live our lives" (Clapp).

What is really alarming is that the biggest segment of our population that is guilty of this self-abuse is in the age group under 44 (like my friend). The problem is particularly bad—and this will possibly impact our society in a negative way for decades to come—among young adults, those in the 18 to 24 age group. A recent survey, conducted by the National Institutes of Health, showed that "at the dawn of the 21st century, young adults were more likely to be smoking, eating badly and sitting on the couch than their counterparts a decade earlier" (Baker).

My friend gets upset with himself that he isn't in shape and his skin still gives him fits, especially in the Texas heat. Every time I show up, I am a reminder of what he *could* be doing.

Notice I did not say *should* be doing. It is his life and his choice. Each time before I leave, I help him outline what he needs to do. We work out a food plan, internal cleansing routine, and a very mild exercise plan.

When I call a couple of weeks later, he either hasn't found the time or has no patience for getting results and gives up "HE IS NOT WILLING TO PAY THE PRICE!"

He, like all of us, has his excuses. Recognize any of the following?

- I will start Monday. Nobody starts a diet (or an exercise program) in the middle of the week.
- Monday's not a good day to start anything new. I am so tired from the weekend.

32

- I have too much pressure at work to start now—after the new manager arrives, things will be better.
- Hey, I don't look (feel) as bad as a lot of people.
- Just one more time! I need to get it out of my system, and I will be ready to change.
- At my age, why bother?
- I've got years to get myself together. I don't have to start today.
- I will wait until after the holidays (vacation, my birthday, etc.)
- I refuse to be controlled by the media's interpretation of what is good and what is bad.
- I want to love myself for who I am.
- I want others to love me for who I am.
- It's all in my genes, anyway. Everybody in my family was fat (had acne, smoked, drank too much, etc.)

I bring this up because we as a society have turned into people who expect magic bullets and miracle pills to "pay the price for us." We don't want to do anything to effect a cure.

As a result, we are paying a far more costly price in terms of the quality of life most of us experience. According to A. H. Mokdad, chief of the Center for Disease Control's (CDC) Behavioral Surveillance Branch, "Americans just haven't changed their behavior enough."

Changing bad habits is not easy, and many of us are not willing to "pay the price." People who study human behavior explain it this way:

33

In the early stages of our unhealthy behavior, we are sociologically introduced to a substance or an activity that gives us immediate positive feelings while masking the realities and responsibilities of everyday life. Through friends, acquaintances, advertising, or [by] just plain accident, we are introduced to things like cigarettes, alcohol, street drugs, pornography, shopping, the advantages of being sick, [unhealthy] food, or even the 'good old' work ethic.

Through the gradual use of these substances or behavior patterns, our biological drives take over and we start to need or even crave this stimulus [to make us feel good]. ("Take Control Now!")

The feeling controls the action. We resist change, refuse to give up our unhealthy habits, to give up our addictions to our unhealthy coping mechanisms, because we don't want to let go of what makes us feel good.

The good news is that healthy habits help us cope as well as unhealthy habits but with positive instead of negative side effects. The only other difference is the time it takes them to work. Shortcuts (bad habits) make us feel good immediately; creating good habits takes time. Bad habits fulfill that desire for that "magic bullet," but the price we pay is continued bad health.

We continue even though, as in the case of acne, for example, the pills and treatments do not work. We get frustrated and angry. We want things the easy way—we do not want to "pay the price" of changing.

However, we are willing to "pay the price" in dollars for what we hope will be an "easy fix." A whole industry, the "cosmeceutical" industry, has been born and thrives on this desire for an easy fix. Cosmeceutical (a word formed from the words "cosmetics" and "pharmaceutical") products are those remedies "marketed as cosmetics that purportedly have biologically active ingredients that affect the user" (Tsao 2004) These products "define a broad gray area where the practice of medicine and the pursuit of vanity meet" (Tsao).

Indeed, Americans spend more than $1.4 billion a year on remedies and treatments for acne—usually with poor results (skinandhealth.com).The over-the-counter and Internet business in acne treatment products is huge.

A website called "Acne-Tratments-Guide.Com" attempts to review some of the claims made by these products. About Derma Cleanse, a popular acne product sold online, Acne-Treatments-Guide says:

According to Zenmed [the company that sells the acne product], Derma Cleanse is a three part system that helps stop acne by working at 'the source,' as well as on the skin's surface. There are just two problems with the . . . system. The treatment does nothing to treat acne at 'the source,' and acne doesn't live at the skin's surface.

Acne-Treatment-Guide goes on to explain that there is nothing in the pill or gel provided in this treatment that has been proven to help cure acne. As for the "gentle wash" included in the Derma Cleanse regimen, Acne-Treatments-Guide cautions us to remember that acne "is NOT caused by dirt. Cleaning your face will not prevent acne, and this is all the [Derma Cleanse] wash does."

Finally, the Guide suggests that "when you consider that the price of this product is almost $100.00, it makes a lot more sense to save the money for another treatment."

Another product researched by Acne-Treatments-Guide is Proactiv Solutions, another acne medication sold on the Internet, which is probably one of the most popular acne remedies of all time. The Proactiv regimen involves a three-part system that exfoliates, cleans, and attacks acne-causing bacteria. Acne websites checked by the Guide found users overwhelmingly dissatisfied with the result they obtained from Proactiv.

The Guide also found that the only ingredient in the Proactiv regimen that has been clinically tested is "a good ole' 2.5% benzoyl peroxide lotion." Since benzyl peroxide is the only ingredient in the product that has some history of effectiveness with acne, the Guide recommends that users purchase it alone:

"The least expensive one [benzyl peroxide product] we've found is for a 60 gram tube of 2.5% benzyl peroxide gel. It [costs] about $18.00, which is a lot less than the $39.95 price for the beginner Proactiv Solutions kit."

Apparently, we are willing to pay hundreds and thousands of dollars on things that don't work in order to avoid changing something we are doing. Now, happily, the methods I include in the book *are* easy.

They really are and they work. Many people who follow this simple routine see results as I did in just three days, most within one week for sure.

There are those who have to do some additional things because the build-up of what is actually causing the acne has been going on for some time. For those of you who have very **resistant** acne, I have included what you need to do to stamp acne out of your life once and for all.

It is easy, but it takes a little work and an open mind. Are you going to be willing to follow the instructions and "pay the small price" for clear skin and much better health and self- esteem?

I am grateful to have helped thousands of folks clear their skin. I have helped them accomplish this from home and without spending thousands of dollars. I have also guided them to additional things to help their lives from the alternative health field even to removing their acne scars without surgery!

Scarring is a major problem associated with chronic acne. Severe acne is particularly troubling because light casts shadows into the scars making them seem deeper than they actually are. Anything that can bring the scarred level of the skin up to the surrounding surface will normalize the appearance.

The usual method for dealing with stubborn acne scars is some form of skin resurfacing, either dermabrasion or laser surgery. According to Stephen W. Perkins, M.D., president of the American Academy of Facial Plastic and

Reconstructive Surgery of the Meridian Plastic Surgery Center of Indianapolis, "Resurfacing is very appealing to people because it is a way of refreshing the skin's surface and getting a new layer of . . . skin."

Dermabrasion is essentially a kind of sanding. Using a motorized burr, the doctor (usually a plastic surgeon) levels out the surrounding surface skin. The new surface of skin will be lighter and smoother than the original surface but will be level to the scarred tissue. As a result, shadows that cause the dark and deep appearance of the scars will be reduced.

Dermabrasion, however, has many unwanted features. First, the initial treatment will result in only a 20% to 40% improvement. Additional treatments over a long period of time may be necessary. At best, dermabrasion will ultimately result in only moderate improvement.

The procedure itself is difficult and uncomfortable. Although the dermabrasion can be done in the surgeon's office, the patient should expect a fairly lengthy healing period.

Prescription pain medication is necessary up to ten days after the surgery. New dressings and ointments must be applied daily until the skin heals. Swelling can last up to two weeks, and even after the skin heals, the surface may appear sunburned for up to six weeks.

Furthermore, dermabrasion is not inexpensive; a complete treatment of the face can cost about $4000. More often than not, the expense is considered cosmetic and not covered by health insurances.

According to Dr. Jean M Loftus, a leading plastic surgeon in the greater Cincinnati area, "Those who expect more from dermabrasion than it can deliver and those who expect deep . . . acne scars will be removed following a few treatments will be disappointed."

Many plastic surgeons prefer laser surgery over dermabrasion, and the popularity of laser surgery is growing. "According to the American Academy of Cosmetic Surgery in Chicago, nearly 170,00 Americans . . . .underwent resurfacing of the face in 1998, up from 138, 891 in 1996—a 64% increase" (Greeley).

Laser surgery involves controlled burning of the affected area with intense light waves. Lasers are popular because they cause little if any bleeding. In fact, the laser "vaporizes superficial layers of facial skin . . . In a sense, the laser procedure creates a fresh surface over which new skin can grow" (Greeley).

However, like dermabrasion, the laser procedure is not without some serious drawbacks. For darker-skinned ethnic groups, this kind of treatment can produce unpredictable and unwanted changes in skin coloration. Other people simply cannot tolerate the lubricants and ointments used. Allergic reactions may occur making the appearance of the skin actually worse.

As with dermabrasion, the initial appearance is difficult for some patients to cope with. Bruising and swelling are common. According to Tina Alster, M.D., director of the Washington Institute of Dermatologic Laser Surgery in Washington, D.C., "[Laser surgery] is not easy in-easy out surgery . . . [Patients] will be holed up in the house for seven to 10 days. They will have a crusty, oozy, bruised, scabbed, raw-appearing face" (quoted in Greeley). As with dermabrasion, laser surgery must be followed up with aftercare that includes frequent changing of soiled dressings.

Alster also points out that laser surgery, while perhaps better than dermabrasion, is not perfect. Laser surgery can produce 50% improvement but, as Alster admits, patients should not expect unflawed skin. "I can't deliver that" (quoted in Greeley).

I have included information on a wonderful way to remove scarring from home without surgery and with the only company I trust to help with acne scarring. For those of you who have the scarring as I did, this information alone is worth thousands in painful dermabraision and laser surgeries.

If I recommend a method, then it has been tried by me and proven to work. Take a good look at my picture in the front of this book. I have had no surgery or dermabraision for my acne or scarring. I eat chocolate and other goodies moderately, and I do not break out.

I have had my acne "handled" for quite sometime now. I know you will find this very valuable to you because you would have to spend ***hundreds of hours researching and hundreds if not thousands of dollars on books and junk*** that do not help you— just as I did all those years—to put all this together.

How much wasted time and money have you already spent? At the encouragement of my friends and family that I have been able to help, I put all of this information together for you because I know what it is like to face this scourge every day.

I have included not just one but a series of methods to help you. Acne can be "sparked" by several bodily functions. Your body though is NOT the problem and acne is not your fault!

Each method has been proven to get results on its own right. Indeed, some are easier than others. I have been fortunate to have good dermatologists confirm my results and to also receive personal confirmation from the many people who have been helped all around the world.

These methods are not crackpot science at work, but truly effective alternative therapies that can clear acne in as little as three days in many individuals like me. For others who continue to have issues, they have been able to route their acne with the other methods I include or by combining several methods together.

I receive daily emails of thanks from satisfied customers for getting this information out to the world. I enjoy all the stories of great successes, and I am sure you have read some of them on our website already.

If I could do it for free, I certainly would! However, websites cost major money to design and maintain. Continuing research also takes time and money.

To get the most out of *Acne Free In 3 Days*, I ask you *read the entire book* before you try any of the recommendations. I share my personal story so you can prepare your mind and get rid of the myths you have picked up about acne.

I want you to dispel the feeling that somehow you are to blame for your breakouts. I also want you to know that my staff and I answer all customer questions and help with the process by staying accessible to you—something no other author does!

You cannot get that from another book! Once you leave the bookstore, you will never hear from that person again. I, on the other hand, try to help all of our clients as much as I can.

That is a 24-hour job in itself, because I care about you and your success! I sincerely want to help you and that is why, if you work all the methods I include and do not get any relief, we offer the refund for those who are willing to pay the price to have clear skin.

If you don't "feel like it" and decide to skip (or not pay the small price), that is certainly up to you. I suggest you put the book up for a while and think on it. People are always amazed that later they suddenly "feel like it."

I have recommended several alternative methods to cure your acne. All have merit and proven results. If one does not work satisfactorily, you should try another. It is important to state here that we have never had someone who really worked the methods and was determined to clear their acne who did not get results—that is a hard fact.

Together we can get your acne calmed down and "cured." You will have to do the work on your side, but I will support you 100%. I expect you to read and follow the directions for any and/or all methods you use.

To gain the most from this book, you must read it in its entirety first. Remember, you need to educate your mind and your body on the real reasons behind your acne, and by doing so, you clear the way for great results.

You can expect me to be there to answer questions and offer support. You will win the battle with your acne! Having gone through what you are struggling through, I am in a good position to share my findings and experience with you. However, legally I must share the following with you:

Disclaimer: "I am not a doctor and I am not intending to treat or cure any disease; I'm simply sharing my personal experience with acne and what I found that worked for me and works for so many others."

Why Me?

It started, as it does for most people, when I was a teenager, a fifteen year old. Like an ugly shadow, it followed me around for the next ten years. It would defy every dermatologist and their expensive prescriptions, treatments with over-the-counter products, ongoing six a.m. antibiotics that created nausea beyond belief, and even Accutaine—the "Miracle Drug."

It would engage me in a fifteen-year war against myself. It was acne, and it was *NOT* my friend. It stole my self-confidence and made me think and feel that there was something wrong with me.

There is no battle as emotionally taxing as one that makes you feel as if your own body is working against you. Your face is what you present to the world—it is your calling card—and *my* card was marked with embarrassing sores and pain. Why me?

So, as I said, when my acne problems started, I was just a teenage guy. I played some sports, which, of course, seemed to make it worse. Acne made me much shyer than I would have otherwise been. "Getting called 'pizza face' doesn't exactly help improve self-image. Academic achievement and personality development suffer. Depression and hopelessness can set in to create a feeling of total inferiority" (Robinson).

45

A recent study conducted by the American Academy of Dermatology (AAD) cited the following as the "invisible" problems of acne: depression, anger, decreased self-esteem, poor body image, social withdrawal, embarrassment, frustration, preoccupation, and even higher rates of unemployment. Unfortunately, the effects are interrelated, and one effect can easily lead to the next, compounding the problems associated with both the physical and emotional health of the acne sufferer (acnenet.com).

Fortunately, I had some good friends and a girlfriend who didn't care about my acne other than how it made me feel. I was in many activities and my acne problem was always right there with me—front and center!

When people looked at me, all I could think was that all they were seeing was the ugly acne on my face. It depressed me and influenced my thoughts and decisions. I was not happy at all, so I tried to find ways to calm it down.

My family and even some of my friends tried to give me all kinds of advice. "Don't eat chocolate," they would say. "Stay away from fish," they would offer. (Easy, I don't like fish!) Everywhere I turned, I found plenty of advice.

Since nearly every adult has "survived" acne, many respond with the advice that nothing can be done but "wait it out." Worse, a lot of different—often contradictory—attitudes are floating around about what works and what doesn't work.

- Wash your skin hard and frequently, for acne is caused by poor hygiene and dirt;
- Washing your skin too hard (or too often) will only make the scarring worse;
- Don't eat french fries and other greasy foods;
- Diet has nothing to do with acne;
- When you start having sex, your acne will clear up (ha!);
- Too much sex will cause acne;
- The wrong kind of sex will cause acne;
- Sunbathing will "dry up" your acne;
- Acne is contagious—you have to "contract" it from someone;
- It's all about heredity and hormones;
- Stress causes acne so don't get stressed (yeah!);
- Seek professional help—let an expert treat you.

However, the acne was still there to greet me each and every morning. I bought and tried every over-the-counter product, and finally I went to several dermatologists. Some were helpful to me but most were not.

One would say it was what I was eating and another would tell me it had nothing to do with that at all. It was bad enough that I was getting conflicting advice from everyone else. Even the 'experts," I was to find out, don't agree! I was frustrated and confused.

I was constantly washing my face and becoming more embarrassed as the cysts and bumps continued their cycle of increasing month after month. Sometimes I would sit for hours with the soap drying on my face hoping to kill the acne, but it did not work.

Once I got so angry and frustrated I slapped my very own face! Deep somewhere inside of me, I felt there was something wrong with me and that my own body was at war with me.

Finally, in the summer of 1983, my mother convinced me to see a new dermatologist. It was my senior year and there were proms to go to, senior pictures to take, and many events to attend.

She wanted me to feel good about this special time in my life. However, it was going to be expensive for us to see this dermatologist because he was very well-known and his office was 30 miles away in another town.

I felt bad because I knew we really did not have the money for doctors. Still, secretly I was excited that I might be able to finally take some pill and be rid of the acne.

So began the years of dermatology visits and thousands of dollars in prescription medicines. My doctor was a good one, and, looking back on it now, I realize he was probably the most honest with me about acne.

Again, he was progressive and well-known. Many people came from three states around to see him. When we arrived at his office that first time, it was very hot.

He was located in a nice new office building that still smelled of carpet and paint. I walked in, signed in, and sat down to wait. Finally, a nurse, or what looked like a nurse, opened a door and called my name.

As I sat in this stark white new patient room, I wondered if he could really help me. I remembered I didn't really like going to doctors.

I felt a familiar tingle, and I scratched a place on my face and it began to bleed. Great! I yanked a paper towel down from the dispenser and quickly dabbed the spot. Then, Dr. Bander walked in.

He was a middle-aged man, slightly overweight, and kind of disheveled looking. His tie was crooked, but he had a nice smile. He started speaking to me in a soft kind of staccato voice, while I stuffed the paper towel in my pocket.

"Well, I am afraid you have two different kinds of acne. You have the surface kind that we can easily help with peeling agents, so I am going to prescribe a lotion for that.

"You also have cystic acne and that can also be called acne vulgaris. Those are deeply infected pores that swell and can cause permanent damage to the collagen under your skin."

He continued. "You see, genetics has done you a great favor in giving you plenty of oil to lubricate your skin. However, at the same time, you have small pores and they become blocked very easily. Thus, the acne on your face."

I said, "Ok," not really being too sure of what he was saying. I just wanted a cure.

His explanation was fairly typical of the best authorities at that time. The development of acne, it was believed, went something like this. During adolescence, hormones stimulate hair growth and oil (sebum) in the skin, especially on the face, arms, neck, and upper torso of the body. In people with acne, the production of scales (keratin) increases faster than the body can shed them (why this happens, is not really understood).

The opening of the hair "follicle" (the built-up oil just under the skin's surface) can become clogged with these extra scales. Certain kinds of bacteria live naturally in the hair, including *Proionbacterium acne (P. acnes)*, the bacterium usually responsible for acne infections. These bacteria take advantage of the blocked hair follicle. They settle in and soon begin to multiple. The hair follicle becomes inflamed and may rupture.

There are numerous systems used to classify acne. The following classification is based upon the severity of the acne:

- **Type 1.** Identified by less than 10 lesions (plugged pores), usually only on the face. (A lesion is a kind of generic term that simply means injury or wound to the skin. In the case of acne, it refers to the plugged oil gland.) These lesions are called "comedones" ("comedo" in the singular) by dermatologists. A comedo can be either a "whitehead" or a "blackhead." A whitehead is a clogged pore that is closed to the surface; a blackhead is open. (The color of a blackhead is not from dirt. It gets its black color from the follicle.)

Type 1 is also identified sometimes with an occasional "papule" (a small, solid bump on the skin) or "pustule" (a papule that contains pus. "Pus" is simply the body's white blood cells that attack the plugged pore and fight infection). A pustule usually forms over a follicle with a hair shaft in the center. (Incidentally, it is the pustule that adolescents are so fond of squeezing or "popping.") With Type 1, there is little or no inflammation and no scarring.

- **Type 2.** Identified by 10 to 25 lesions on face and trunk of the body. Whiteheads and blackheads are more numerous. Some inflammation and mild scarring.

- **Type 3.** Identified by numerous comedones, papules, and pustules, spreading to back, chest, shoulders. An occasional "cyst" (a sac-like lesion filled with liquid or semi-liquid, larger than the pustule and severely inflamed) or "nodule" (a firm, severe lesion that extends into the deep layers of the skin) may appear. Moderate scarring.

- **Type 4.** Identified by numerous large cysts and nodules on face, neck, upper trunk. Severe scarring.

The above system provides some good terms that are useful in the discussion of acne. However, like many of the classification systems, it relies on the observation of the individual doctor. Since this observation is subjective, changing from person to person, it isn't terribly useful.

My doctor's explanation of acne would be what I believed about the nature of acne for many years to come.

It would be another ten years before I would discover that acne comes from a completely different source altogether and that too much oil and small pores are not the problem.

"So what do I do now, Doctor?" I asked. He detailed a routine of antibiotics. He said he was glad I was older because they would not turn my teeth yellow! Yellow teeth and discoloration of the skin are side effects of antibiotics at a young age.

I didn't know it then, but those very antibiotics that were supposed to help quell the infection were going to set me up for severe adult acne problems later on. "You understand and feel ok with what we are going to do?" he asked.

"Sure, fine with me." I lied. I paid my $300.00, picked up the prescription notes, and left. I then began the normal routine that most of us go through.

Dr. Bander prescribed tetracycline, an antibiotic, and I would be taking three pills in the morning at about 6 a.m., so they could dissolve before breakfast. Tetracycline is the antibiotic most often prescribed for acne. In fact, it is prescribed so often and for so many problems that it is sometimes referred to as the "house call" antibiotic.

Then I was to apply this lotion called Persa-gel, a 10% solution of benzyl peroxide. Benzyl peroxide, I was to find out, was the most frequently used "topical" (applied to the surface of the skin) treatment. Dr. Bander, apparently, was on the cutting edge of acne biomedicine.

The best thing about benzoyl peroxide is that it has few of the side effects that seem to be associated with almost all acne treatments. It is also inexpensive and, in the long run, is probably just as useful (or useless) as the more sophisticated "designer" antibiotics and other drugs.

The worst side effect, and the one most often experienced by acne sufferers, is a redness or dryness of the skin.

The benzyl peroxide would dry up my skin and cause it to exfoliate. "Exfoliation" is the peeling of skin, which is supposed to unplug pores and remove dead skin. As I read the prescription packages, I remember my conversation with him. "It will take about six weeks to get this calmed down. Then we will give you an antibody shot with a needle in the larger cysts to limit scarring, which you already have some."

I replied hastily, "Great...I have scars?" I was really worried.

Dr. Bander then said, "Look on the bright side...with your skin being oily, you will never have to worry about a lot of wrinkles!" At 18 I was not worried about wrinkles, but the thought of scarring had not occurred to me, and it terrified me.

I followed the routine for six weeks, until my next visit. The six a.m. dose of the tetracycline was awful. Anyone who has ever taken antibiotics on an empty stomach, as I had to do, knows the nausea is terrible. My education in antibiotics was just beginning. Nausea is, in fact, a common side effect with most antibiotics:

Antibiotics cause gastrointestinal reactions by direct irritation of the mucous membrane, destruction of normal, natural bacterial flora or by creating bacterial overgrowth of abnormal forms. Antibiotics eliminate organism from the normal flora of the skin, oral and genitor-urinary mucosa and promote growth of drug-resistant organisms. (tuberose.com)

In effect, this means that "antibiotics in our bodies cannot tell the cops from the robbers" (tuberose.com). They kill bad bacteria, but they also kill the millions of good bacteria (*microflora*) that live naturally in our bodies, including in our intestines—bacteria that, among other things, help us digest the food we eat. When these friendly bacteria are killed, food cannot digest and we become sick. These good bacteria are also useful for digesting and destroying yeast cells that can cause several different kinds of yeast infections in the body.

Our standard dictionary will tell us that antibiotics are "substances having the power to arrest or kill microorganisms called germs" (tuberose.com).

However, "medical dictionaries define 'antibiotics' as a chemical substance produced by a microorganism, which kill other microorganisms" (tuberose.com). It probably wouldn't have stopped me from taking the tetracycline— but still, it is interesting to note that the word "antibody" actually means *against life*!

I applied the prescription gel as directed, and it burned a little. Then, off I went to school. I felt pretty good, knowing my acne problem was being treated. Of course, nothing noticeable happened for about two weeks, except my skin was very dull looking and flaky. I noticed it also bled very easily.

Then one day, it happened. I was sitting in my class when I felt something wet begin to trickle down my left cheek. I reached up. A place on my face had opened up, and a stream of clear liquid was pouring out.

It was so gross, and I was so embarrassed! I had to ask to leave. In the restroom, I quickly grabbed brown paper towels that were not absorbing anything. I grabbed the toilet paper and finally the great Niagara Falls on my face stopped.

As soon as I got home, I made a phone call to the dermatologist. He explained to me that it could happen from time to time, so I better carry some tissues with me. This was crazy!

What he didn't tell me (my education was continuing) was that using antibiotics can actually increase the severity and number of infections over time.

In fact, "the inappropriate use of an antibiotic can result in the appearance of resistant strains of bacteria . . ." (Simmons). Essentially, what this means is that the bacteria that survive the steady bombardment of antibiotics have "figured out" a way to "outsmart" the antibiotic. These "smarter" and stronger germs reproduce leaving the antibiotic useless, at least at its original strength.

The human body has been fighting off bacteria for about 100,000 generations—at least until the late 1930s and early 1940s when antibiotics were developed—without the use of antibiotics:

Humans and other animals don't produce antibiotics, nor do they need to, if their endocrine, immune, and nervous systems have the mineral, vitamin, protein, and enzyme substances found in foods gown on mineral-rich soil. Armed with these tools, the Earth's highest forms of life— humans and animals—are well equipped to fight the Earth's lowest forms of life, bacteria and fungi. (tuberose.com)

The overuse of antibiotics prevents the body's natural systems from doing the jobs they had done for thousands of years. According to Dr W. Eugene Sanders, associate Professor of Medicine and Microbiology at the University of Florida, College of Medicine, "there was a time when there was so much penicillin used on hospital wards that one could detect minute organisms of penicillin in the air" (tuberose.com).

Penicillin, the drug that began the antibiotics era, was believed to be the answer to infectious diseases that have plagued mankind for centuries. However, Alexander Fleming, the scientist who discovered penicillin, warned against the dangers of its overuse. The drug was introduced to the public in 1944; by 1946, within two years of its introduction, 14 percent of the bacteria that penicillin initially killed proved to be resistant to it. By 1959, 59 percent showed a resistance (Nelson).

What was true of penicillin, proved to be true for all antibiotics. Streptomycin, introduced to the public in 1945, faced its first resistance in 1959; Erythromycin, introduced in 1952, began to fail in 1988; and Tetracycline began to lose its war against bacteria in 1953, just five years after its introduction to the public (tnguyen2 2005). The hard fact remains that "resistance is a natural evolutionary response that humans cannot stop" (tnguyen 2).

"Bacteria resistant (sic) to antibiotics is a rapidly emerging problem with potentially disastrous consequences" (Antibiotics!) Today the bacteria that cause bacterial pneumonia, ear infections, meningitis, and gonorrhea, as well as most "staph" (*staphylococcus*) infections have developed at least some resistance to penicillin, which used to be used as the antibiotic of choice against each of these diseases.

The resistance of the acne bacteria (*P.acnes*) to oral antibiotics was first recognized in the late 1970s. This resistance is especially noted with the use of the antibiotics erythromycin and tetracycline, the two antibiotics most used in the treatment of acne.

As one member of the American College of Physicians put it, "As antibiotic use and costs have soared (to $15 billion per year in the United States alone), these miracle drugs of the 1940s are becoming the dismal failures of the new millennium" (Fryhofer 2005).

After I graduated from high school, my acne calmed a little, but I had breakouts of varying degrees ongoing for the next year. However, this time I was learning to live with it.

Sometimes though the breakouts were as bad as when I was 17. When I went off to college to study broadcasting and film, my acne became a real world problem. The heavy theatrical make up made it worse since my skin could not breathe. Doctors are not in complete agreement on the use of make-up over acne, but most agree that excessive use of make-up—such as actors might use—does make the condition worse.

So, the off and on visits to my dermatologist continued. As I became more successful, I began to get small parts in films and on television. I even got an agent named Peggy Taylor, who was like a second mother to me.

She made it clear that, for me to be really successful, I was going to have to get my acne under control. As Dr. Fredrick Work, a plastic and reconstructive surgeon in Atlantic explains it, "[Even before] you can open your mouth to express yourself, people have already formed an opinion about who you are based on your looks."

Peggy was right. I guess I already knew that casting directors, whose job it is to consider audiences' responses to actors, would reject me, at least subconsciously, even before I had a chance to audition. To put it bluntly, the audience wouldn't get beyond their own prejudices about acne no matter how good an actor I was. There it was once more—my acne standing in my way. Depressed, I told her I would do it somehow.

Desperate again, I called Dr. Bander and explained my dilemma. When I called, he had good news. He asked me to try a new prescription product named Accutane (brand name for isotretinoin), the expensive and strong drug by Roche. Little did I know at the time—little did anyone know at the time—Accutane would become one of the most popular and controversial drugs in the history of the pharmaceutical industry.

Accutane, which was introduced to the public as an acne "wonder drug" in 1982, is not an antibiotic. Rather, it is chemically related to vitamin A. It is still, today, the strongest medication prescribed by doctors for the treatment of acne. It is the medication most dermatologists regard as the drug of "last resort," used only for those patients whose acne is very severe and has proven resistant to topical treatments (including both over-the-counter creams and astringents and prescription ointments and creams) and to antibiotics (specifically, tetracycline and erythromycin, the two most often prescribed antibiotics for acne).

It was a very new drug and required me to have biweekly blood testing to make sure it did not adversely affect my liver. I was told that aside from some unpleasant side effects, Accutane helped to reduce the chances of scars and pox marks by putting your acne into remission.

Theoretically, Accutane works against acne by stopping skin pores from producing sebum [oil]. When sebum production slows or stops, there is no longer any way for the acne causing bacteria to grow, because . . . the bacteria grow in the sebum produced in the skin. No more sebum = no more acne. (Acne-Treatments-guide.com)

Champions of Accutane were claiming that it was successful in treating even the most stubborn cases of acne, specifically those cases that had proven to be resistant to antibiotics. According to the experts, a treatment session would last 15 to 20 weeks at most; and that would be it—I'd never experience acne again.

It seemed to me to be the answer to a prayer, the "wonder drug" (the "magic bullet") that would finally rid me of this scourge.

I was willing to do ***anything*** to make it better. The myth that guys do not care about their appearance is a big lie. I cared and I wanted it gone, period.

A week later, I began taking the Accutane. At least it did not make me sick to my stomach the way the antibiotics had. Two weeks passed, and I began to get very dry skin.

My face, however, was not as inflamed. Could it be it was working? A week later, I went for my biweekly blood test. I had to fast for 12 hours before they could do the test to determine if my lipids and liver were functioning properly. I took the blood test and got the all-clear.

After six weeks, my skin looked really good. No new cysts had appeared, and my little red marks looked better. I was very happy with the progress. As happy as I was, I soon would find out that taking this drug had its price. I had a few scars I had never noticed because my face was always so red from the acne. Still, I was happy—no, I was ecstatic—it was finally gone. I was cured!

Accutane has well-known side effects. Dry skin and some joint pain are normal. I had a mild case of each, but then something horrific happened. I was at an event for my college.

I finished the speech I had prepared for that day and confidently strode down the steps into the auditorium. I reached up to wipe the damp sweat from my forehead and felt a strange sensation on my left brow.

My entire eyebrow had completely come off on my fingers!

My girlfriend freaked, and we rushed to the bathroom. I was horrified and would not even touch the right side of my face.

She quickly stenciled one on for me with her eyebrow pencil, so I would not stand out. Hair loss associated with Accutane was common when I took it. Over the next several months, my hair would fall out in clumps. To me this was worse than acne itself.

Other side effects of Accutane—some of them simply bothersome but some of them very serious—were becoming known to the public. The list of suspected or confirmed side effects was pretty long:

- chapped lips
- dry skin
- conjunctivitis ("pink eye")
- itching
- nausea, vomiting
- liver disease
- dry nasal passage
- nose bleed
- headaches
- sensitive skin around body openings (mouth, nose, anus, etc.)
- dry eyes
- hair loss

(Acne-Treatment-Guide.com)

I was assured my hair would grow back, and eventually it did. I took the drug for six horrific months, and then it was time to stop. My skin and face were clear of the acne, and my eyebrow had grown back, and it did appear the acne was gone for good. My acne was in "remission."

So, I really felt, overall, Accutane was wonderful (except for those horrific side effects). After finishing college, I moved on into my profession. For the next two years, I was able to enjoy a life with clear skin.

Then one morning I got up like normal to go to work. As I looked into the mirror, I could not believe what I saw. With no warning whatsoever, my face was completely covered in new acne breakouts. I was shocked and in disbelief; how could this be? It was back!

At first, I was sure I must have been having an allergic reaction. It had to be; there could be no other explanation. I quickly made an appointment to see a top dermatologist in the city in which I was then living.

Her name was Carol, and I counted down the days to get in to see her. In the meantime, I tried all my old ways of calming my acne down. Of course, like before, they did nothing.

If it had caused frustration and grief in the past, it was really irritating me even worse now. I was not in school anymore, and I was an executive!

I stood before the mirror in unspeakable outrage as the scourge returned. I washed and washed my face over and over again. (Old ways of reacting to my acne were coming to the fore). It was not good.

It was a Tuesday afternoon, and I sat very impatiently in the doctor's waiting room—this time in a high rise. Finally, I was called and I went in. Carol was pleasant enough but not at all like Dr. Bander.

I wasn't sure what I was expecting. She told me to relax and explained I was not having an allergic reaction. "Acne tends to return in many Accutane patients." I remembered the horrific six months during which I took the drug, hoping that, at last, I had found an end to this hell once and for all.

Accutane, the "wonder drug" for the treatment of acne, was beginning to seem a little less wonderful to me.

She also quickly ran down the familiar drill. "Acne has nothing to do with food; you will need to begin taking antibiotics again." I felt myself begin sinking into the hard table I sat on. "Antibiotics?" I muttered.

I told her antibiotics had never worked for me and asked, "Why couldn't I take the Accutane again?" She quickly told me the drug was "too harsh" and she "didn't believe in it."

Carol, as it turned out, wasn't alone in her condemnation of Accutane. Few drugs have been so hotly discussed in the media and by professionals alike. For a while the Food and Drug Administration (FDA) considered pulling it off the market. The side effects were many, and the suspicions about the drug's "harsh" side effects were being debated everywhere.

Over the years, it has become one of the most tightly regulated drugs sold.

To be able to prescribe this medication, a doctor must be a registered member of the manufacturer's System to Manage Accutane-Related Teratogenicity (SMART) program. The SMART program was developed in conjunction with the U.S. Food and Drug Administration

(FDA) to . . . educate patients to [among other things] the possible adverse effects [of the drug]. (Feldman et al. 2004)

Eventually, even more serious concerns were being raised. Accutane was found to be associated with high percentages of several different kinds of birth defects—including mental retardation and physical malformations—in babies whose mothers were taking the drug. Women of child-bearing age who are considering taking the drug have to be given both spoken and written warnings about the importance of using birth control while on the drug. Two negative pregnancy urine tests are required before Accutane is prescribed; pregnancy status is checked at monthly visits to the doctor.

Furthermore, women of child-bearing age are required to sign a form noting that they have been informed of the following:

- Accutane is a powerful "last resort" treatment for acne;
- You must not take Accutane if you are pregnant or may become pregnant during your treatment;
- If you get pregnant while taking Accutane, your baby will be at high risk for birth defects;
- If you take Accutane, you must use at least one effective birth control form (two are recommended) one month before the start of treatment through one month after the end of treatment;

- You must test negative for pregnancy within two weeks before starting Accutane, and you must start Accutane on the second or third day of your menstrual period;
- You may participate in a program that includes an initial free pregnancy test and birth control counseling session;
- If you become pregnant, you must immediately stop taking Accutane and see your doctor;
- You have read and understood the Accutane patient brochure and asked your doctor any questions you had;
- You are not currently pregnant and do not plant to become pregnant for at least 30 days after you finish taking Accutane;
- You have been invited to participate in a survey of women being treated with Accutane. ("Side Effects")

Since its introduction to the public in 1982, isotretinoin (Accutane) has been linked to psychiatric disorders such as depression and suicide. Lawyers and parents have implicated the drug in the hospitalizations and suicides of over 200 teenagers in the United States. Douglas Bremner of the Emory University School of Medicine suggests that doctors ask their patients about depression and suicidal thoughts before prescribing the medication to "ensure the well-being of their patients" (2005).

Of course, Carol was the expert not me. She continued to explain, "A lot of my patients have taken Accutane, and the remission never lasts more than a year or so." Her words were stinging.

She certainly thought she was the expert. I picked up the prescription, paid my bill, and left. I was frustrated and pissed off as I marched back out into the hot Texas sun.

That night I had dinner with a good friend named Katie. My friend was into holistic therapies and stuff I did not understand at the time. After about an hour of me venting over our drinks, she asked me if I had tried any herbal approaches.

"Don't you think you should at least look into it?" she asked. I didn't answer. "Chris, lots of people are finding alternative ways to combat things like acne that the AMA doesn't believe in."

At the time, I associated herbal treatments and remedies, as well as all kinds of alternative medical practices, with incense and strobe lights and countercultural hippies and potheads and other seedy and slightly illegal activities. I imagined eighteenth-century opium dens in faraway Chinese ports-of-call or nineteenth-century traveling medicine shows selling snake oil to gullible cowboys or laudanum to frustrated pioneer women. At the very least I didn't want to harm myself; I also didn't want to feel foolish or desperate for "buying into" such nonsense.

I assumed, the way most of us do I guess, that holistic healthcare was simply the opposite of traditional, proven healthcare, what is sometimes called "allopathy" or "mainstream" medicine. In essence, holistic medicine, I believed, was quackery.

I did not know that while alternative medicine in the United States often developed apart from conventional approaches, most cultures—about 80% of the world according to the World Health Organization—recognize the legitimacy of the holistic tradition. In fact, many traditional remedies and practices were first considered nontraditional. I knew that herbal medicine predated traditional medicine, that the Egyptians and the Greeks and Romans used herbs.

Perhaps this knowledge made me regard nontraditional medicine as not only alternative medicine but as primitive medicine. And I wanted no part of that.

Conventional medicine, I would learn, is simply medicine practiced by an M.D. and allied health personnel: registered nurses, pharmacists, and therapists. However, conventional medicine differs in another important way from alternative medicine: while the traditional approach seeks primarily to get rid of symptoms and to heal the individual diseased or broken organ, the holistic approach, as the name indicates, seeks to involve the whole person (mind, body, and spirit).

Another important aspect of holistic healing that I was to discover was the emphasis that it places upon balance in the organism. Ancient cultures and so-called primitive cultures have always recognized the need for balance.

The ancient Greek culture—to whom our own culture owes so many of our cherished traditions—recognized the need for balance in its description of the four "humors" or energies of the body. The Greeks picked up many of the traditions of the people whom they conquered. Among these traditions was the belief that herbs in some way affected the balance of these four energies or properties (humors): air, water, earth, and fire. When these properties were out of balance, the individual experienced illness. Herbs were used and evaluated according to their ability to reestablish a balance in the body's humors.

A similar approach has been used for centuries in Traditional Chinese Medicine (TCM).

TCM is based on a concept of balanced qi (pronounced 'chee'), or vital energy, that is believed to flow throughout the body. Qi is proposed to regulate a person's spiritual, emotional, mental, and physical balance and to be influenced by the opposing forces of yin (negative energy) and yang (positive energy). Disease . . . results from the flow of qi being disrupted and yin and yang becoming imbalanced. (National Institutes of Health, D156).

While alternative medicine as we know it in the United States today may not rely on "humors," "qi," and "yin and yang," it does carry with it this emphasis upon balance as necessary for good health. In most holistic approaches, the body is regarded as capable of its own curative powers once it is put back into a balanced state.

One leader in the holistic community put it this way: "Your body has a BLUEPRINT, a SCHEMATIC of what perfect health is and it is constantly trying to achieve this perfect health for you, all that goes wrong is that you get in the way of this natural process" (Schulze).

"Alternative approaches work," my friend Katie explained. "I personally don't see why you should ignore something that might be able to help you. Do you want to continue to suffer with your skin? You're obviously not happy."

I told her no I wasn't happy, and I would be willing to try anything because I knew the antibiotics were not going to work. She directed me to an herbalist in a nearby town, and I told her I would at least check it out.

I was desperate not to go back to my old days of skin problems. There are a few times in your life when you can look back in retrospect and say that a decision you made was a true turning point in your life. My decision to go to the herbalist certainly turned out to be one for me.

As I sat in bumper-to-bumper traffic in 100 degree Texas heat, I stared at the directions to the herbal place she had given me on the back of a cocktail napkin. I had called them to make sure they were still open, and I hoped I'd make it before they closed.

I had not asked how *late* they stayed open and the radio announcer was saying there was an accident. "Great," I thought. Maybe this just isn't meant to be.

I found another station playing music, pulled my sunglasses down my nose, and leaned my head back on my headrest and waited.

Twenty minutes later, the accident cleared, and I was on my way again. It was after 6 p.m.

"Man, they are going to be closed," I murmured as I pulled into the small parking lot. I had arrived at "Herbals—Are—You," and found I had an hour left according to the sign on the door.

There was a "Ya'll come on in" wooden sign with little chimes hanging on the door. They clanked instead of chiming as I opened it, and a smell of incense hit my nose. "Oh brother," I thought. "Bet herbs aren't all they sell here."

"May I be of some assistance?" an invisible voice asked. I looked around but didn't see anyone. "Uh, yeah, my name is Chris and I called earlier?" There was silence.

I peered behind the sales counter. "Oh yes!" came a voice directly behind me. Startled, I turned around.

That's when I first saw Mary Campbell, the owner and only employee of the shop. Once again, images of strobe lights and the 1960s flashed through my mind. Mary, I initially decided, was a hippie re-tread, a throwback to the days of sex, drugs, and rock-n-roll. What was I doing here, I asked myself. For a moment I considered turning around and getting the heck out of there. I felt foolish and gullible, even pathetic.

Mary Campbell, I soon found out, was a 60-something lady who looked like she was 40. She had opened the store about 20 years ago and had seen and talked to people about every kind of malady.

She had lived and worked as an herbalist for most of her life. She wore her very red hair piled not so neatly on top of her head, which seemed too big for her body.

Her glasses made her eyes look like an owl's eyes and gave her the appearance of being very wise. "Poor eyesight," she said, as if reading my mind. "You know, from reading all these labels and bottles." Her accent was thick but sweet. Old enough to be my grandmother, Mary had that intuitive ability that mothers have with their children. If she asks to read my palm, I thought to myself, I'm out of here!

I wanted nothing more than to end the awkwardness of the situation. "I'm sorry, but I really don't have a lot of time," I lied. "All I need is something to help me clear up this acne." I was feeling uncomfortable, and I was now growing more anxious to leave. I was pretty sure this place was not for me.

My friend Katie was probably having a good laugh about now. Still, I had tried so many treatments and remedies; I supposed this one couldn't be any more ridiculous than some of the others I had tried over the years. One bad remedy was as good (or bad) as the next, I decided. I would see this one through to the end, too. "Do you think you can help me?" I asked sheepishly.

"Well, Sweetie, that's what I'm here for! Katie has already told me most of what you have been through. It's sad, but this happens to many people.

"The drugs just do not work, and they do not know what to do. I have already made a list of what you will need." She handed me a used paper receipt on which she had listed what I needed (pretty unprofessional, I thought skeptically).

Mary took the time to go through every herb that helps the skin and acne. She talked about the body and how acne and skin conditions in general were getting worse. Acne was becoming another of the so-called "diseases of affluence," those noncommunicable (noncontagious) diseases linked to a modern and affluent lifestyle (I thought of my overweight friend in Dallas and his unwillingness to "pay the price" to get into shape). Furthermore, these "diseases of affluence" are largely preventable. In fact, bad habits—poor diet, lack of exercise, smoking—were now responsible for one-third of all deaths in the United States.

I recalled my dermatologist saying something like that, and now I wished I had paid more attention. Mary continued to describe how diet does play a role, and that sugar and soft drinks were really hard on the body and skin.

Most people, I believe, know that sugars and soft drinks especially, have little nutritional value, that they are essentially empty calories. Unfortunately, sugars (and sugar substitutes) are not simply neutral: they are actually harmful and are a leading cause of poor health in affluent cultures, particularly in the United States.

Because most Americans eat their own weight in sugar every year, they are susceptible to a number of diseases and maladies associated with the imbalance of proper nutrients and hormones in the body. When we flood our body with too much sugar (almost any sugary snack will do this), our body is overwhelmed and cannot maintain the proper balance of sugar (glucose) in the blood. The results of too much refined (white) sugar include:

- anxiety and panic attacks
- eating disorders including bulimia and anorexia nervosa
- menstrual dysfunctions including mood swings and depression
- dental diseases, especially tooth decay
- low energy and hypoglycemia
- addictions (both of food and drugs, including cigarettes)
- mineral and vitamin depletions, especially of the B vitamins
- diabetes
- candida (yeast) infections (candida feeds on sugar)
- constipation
- obesity

(Later in this chapter, we will also see how sugar contributes to the development of acne.)

If sugar is bad, sugary soft drinks are worse, especially colas and other dark drinks. Russell J. Martino, Ph.D., puts it this way: "Of all the things I can think of that can inflict maximum damage on your health, the regular consumption of soft drinks, **regular or diet** (emphasis added), is one of the most powerful."

Have you ever read the label on a can of Coke or Dr. Pepper?

Forget about the fact that these drinks contain about 10 teaspoons of sugar per 12-ounce can. Note instead that one of the other main ingredients of all dark-colored soft drinks is phosphoric acid!

According to Dr. Martino, "Drinking down a tall, cool glass of phosphoric acid laced with sugar is just a little less bad for you than gulping down a bottle of toilet bowl cleaner!"

Nonetheless, our bodies constantly fight to return to a balanced state no matter what we pour down our throats. The phosphoric acid that is contained in these dark beverages is somewhat neutralized by the calcium in our bodies. Guess where the body goes for its supply of calcium to combat all that phosphoric acid?

Yeah, our bones are made of calcium, more than enough to balance out even the most addictive soft drink consumption. The only problem is that depleting our bones of calcium leaves them brittle and weak. This danger is particularly great for women of menopausal or post-menopausal age.

If you have to drink sugary soft drinks, avoid the dark ones, the ones with phosphoric acid.

Always read the content label, too—good advice for everything you eat and drink. Do some research; know what you are putting into your body. Don't trust manufacturers or the government to know what is best for you. It is your body.

Mary also talked about how material and debris pile up in the lower intestines and make havoc with the body's ability to clean out toxins.

It's probably not one of those problems that most of us want to talk about, but constipation—difficult or infrequent bowel movements resulting from prolonged bowel transit times (the time it takes food to be digested and then eliminated from the body)—is a potentially serious threat to good health and a leading cause of chronic and serious diseases in the human organism, particularly in America. "Americans have the highest incidence of colon-rectal cancer of any nation in the world, and it is now killing more Americans than ever before in history" (Shirley's Wellness Café 2005). The average American will have "2-4 bowel movements a week, coming up 70,000 bowel movements short in their life time" (Shulze).

The gastrointestinal tract (GIT) is an incredibly sensitive and complex system. Most of the actual digestion occurs in the small intestines; here most of the body's nutrients are absorbed from the food we eat. After passing through the small intestines, the remaining waste material passes into the five-foot long large intestines (colon). In the colon, water is extracted and absorbed through the intestine wall; the longer the bowel stays in the colon (the slower the transit time), the harder the bowel becomes.

As far back as the 4th century B.C., the Greek physician Hippocrates acknowledged the importance of the intestines when he stated that "Death begins in the bowels." It is the second largest organ in the body (second only to the human skin) and is the home of billions of intestinal microflora (good bacteria that help our food digest properly).

Over the typical lifespan, a staggering 60 tons of food will pass through the intestines (Hawrelak 2004).

Mary went on to explain how the use of antibiotics made things worse.

"Not only do the antibiotics kill good bacteria, they also kill the naturally occurring bacteria that keep yeast and germs at a minimum."

Substances such as antibiotics and steroids also provide the opportunity for bad bacteria to enter and grow in our systems. (As pointed out earlier, antibiotics are equal opportunity killers. Stupid, they kill good bacteria—such as the bacteria that grow naturally in our guts and keep yeast in check— as well as bad bacteria.) "Alterations in the bowel flora and its activities are now believed to be contributing factors to many chronic . . . diseases" (Hawreiak).

"In the nineteenth century, . . William Harvey Kellogg, of Kellogg's cereal fame, wrote extensively of the dangers of 'autointoxication' purportedly caused by inadequate elimination" (EHC.com 2003). With longer bowel transit times, "the intestinal contents may harden and a person may have difficulty or even pain during elimination."

In severe cases, the colon walls can become lined with layers of fecal matter imbedded in toxic mucus, which can take on the consistency of hard rubber" (DigestivePlus 2005). (If you want to see some really disgusting but convincing pictures, see HPS-Online.com, but be prepared for what you will see!) When this situation occurs, putrefied waste products stay in the intestine longer, and toxins can actually enter the blood stream and find their way into and through other organs of the body (including the skin). This phenomenon is known as "bowel toxemia" or "autointoxication," which means "self-poisoning." In effect, the body poisons itself with its own toxins.

"You see," Mary explained, "when you take antibiotics, especially long term as you have, the balance in your bowel is put off kilter and the Candia yeast goes crazy."

Medical science and many naturalists know this is associated with all kinds of problems from athlete's foot to the yeast infections women get."

Candida albicans, the most common yeast found in the human body and the cause of most so-called yeast infections includes the following:

- diaper rash
- vaginal yeast infection
- certain kinds of diarrhea
- yeast infection of the breast
- thrush

The two most common kinds of yeast infections are the persistent vaginal yeast infections, experienced by two out every three women, and oral yeast infection, also known as "thrush."

Candida albicans is commonly found in the vagina, the colon, and on the skin. It is a part of the natural "community," the millions of organisms that live in and on our bodies.

All yeasts are, in fact, a kind of fungus, which exist naturally as single-celled organisms in humans.

Yeasts are not inherently pathological, that is, they do not naturally cause a normally healthy body any harm. In fact, in a healthy body, when Candida is in balance, it helps our immune system by controlling bacterial growth. Yeast and bacteria are in constant competition for the same space; when antibiotics kill off bacteria, both good and bad, Candida flourishes.

Candida becomes a problem only when—in a body whose system is not in balance—their numbers are no longer kept in check. According to Tom Volk, an expert on fungi,

Some alteration of the host's . . . defenses, physiology, or normal flora must take place before colonization [of Candida], infection, and disease production can take place. This phenomenon is known as "Candida overgrowth." (1999)

Candida overgrowth can produce toxins (poisons) that are associated with many diseases and health-related problems:

- allergies
- chemical sensitivities (a marked distaste for car exhaust, . . [and] ammonia-based cleaners
- chronic fatigue syndrome
- digestive problems, weak digestion, poor nutrient assimilation
- emotional problems
- food cravings, food allergies
- gall bladder problems
- immune system problems
- thyroid problems
- viral infections
- unexplained weight loss
- skin problems

Candida produces an alcohol that contributes or causes most of these problems. Ethanol, the alcohol, intoxicates (poisons) the blood. The yeast grows unchecked if it has an abundant food source. The food source that yeast grows best in is—as any good cook knows—is sugar.

Remember all those sugary foods and soft drinks?

I sat there quietly and continued to listen.

"You have heard of infants having problems with ear infections, right?"

"Sure," I said, wondering where she was going with it. "Well, they almost always get a bad case of thrush, the white coating on the tongue and throat, when they have been on the antibiotics too long.

"All of this is from the yeast or Candida that gets out of control."

"Okay," I said.

She continued. "When Candida Albicans gets out of control and is more prevalent, the good bacteria in your body produce too much toxins for your body to get rid of.

"These toxins can cause allergic reactions to food, and more often than not, they are behind the infections that acne is associated with." She rested her case.

"Well, but my doctors told me it was because my skin is too oily and my pores are too small." I countered.

She looked me straight in the eye. "Chris, your body knows what it is doing. You are not the problem! The combination of what you eat every day and the antibiotics have created this problem. I bet you just love sugar and cokes right?"

"Of course I do; who doesn't?" I was feeling a little defensive. I could remember that whenever I had a regular coke or dark soft drink, I could almost see my skin getting worse in an hour or so. I had shrugged it off as coincidence since my dermatologists said it was not food that caused the breakouts.

"Exactly!" she said. "Many people with Candida infections are very addicted to sugary snacks and things. Candida is yeast, and yeast needs sugar to grow! The problem is made worse by the fact that yeast infections may actually cause a craving for sugar. High blood sugar and an out of balance bowel create a perfect environment for this sort of thing. I see it all the time."

"You will need to replace the naturally occurring bacteria that are missing in your system," she smiled.

"But how can I do that?" I asked her.

"Well, the good news is you can take it in pill form. It is called 'acidophilus b.' and you will be taking it at the same time you cut out all the sugar you can."

 Acidophilus b. (*Lactobacillus acidophilus*) is a type of "friendly" bacteria, what is sometimes referred to a "probiotic" (notice the contrast to the word "antibiotic"). Many yogurts contain acidophilus, but, unfortunately, yogurt usually contains some form of sugar or fruit, too— to make it tastier. We don't want that.

"In addition, you will be taking garlic to help kill off the Candida infection."

82

I never dreamed that garlic was good for anything other than making Italian food delicious and for warding off vampires. Once again, I was to discover the healthy benefit of herbs that have been used by mankind for thousands of years.

Garlic, no doubt, would be on every herbalist's list as the number one most useful herb. It has been cultivated by humans for medicinal and dietary uses longer than any other herb. It has been used by more people in more countries on more continents than any other herb. More important, it has proven to be the most versatile of all herbs.

If it were not for its somewhat potent sulfuric smell (garlic is a good source of sulfur and selenium), garlic would be perfect. In fact, legend has it that someone who rubs garlic on the soles of his feet will exhale the odor from his lungs in just a few short hours!

Owing, perhaps, to its pungent smell, garlic is famous in myths as a defense from vampires and other dark creatures of the underworld. The ancient Greeks who had recently eaten garlic were not allowed into the holy temples. Such an action was considered an affront to the gods.

Garlic is mentioned in the Old Testament as a sustaining staple in the diet of Moses' people as they fled Egypt. The Egyptians themselves used it; legend tells us that the builders of the pyramids used it to increase their stamina as they built their great structures. Soldiers of ancient Rome consumed it for courage, and many Native American tribes cultivated it for its medicinal properties.

Lepers in Asia were once treated with a paste made from the garlic bulb.

During World War I, garlic was used as an antiseptic. The raw juice of the garlic bulb was squeezed onto Sphagnum moss, which was applied as a kind of bandage to a wound. It apparently hastened the healing process and prevented infections. Doctors believe thousands of lives were saved using this ancient herb (Grieve).

Early travel journals report that peasants in Siberia and farmers along the Mediterranean Sea used it in their dishes. Even Shakespeare, who regarded garlic-eaters as vulgar (comparable today, perhaps, to people who dip chewing tobacco) wrote about it in his play *Coriolanus*.

An ancient Moslem legend says it best:

When Satan stepped out from the Garden of Eden after the fall of man, garlic sprang up from the spot where he placed his left foot, and Onion [a close cousin to garlic] from that where his right foot touched. (Quoted in Grieve)

"Kill off? How does garlic kill off yeast?" This was beginning to sound like a lot of work to me, and expensive.

"It is easy and very inexpensive!" she said once again, seeming to read my mind. "I have the tablets you will need right here, and you will start with a three-day fruit cleanse to clean out all the built up debris in your bowel. After that you will begin with these supplements and NO SUGAR!" She was matter of fact.

"Many people have their acne completely clear up after they do the three-day fast," she added.

"Really? In three days? How is that possible?" I was incredulous now.

Still a little skeptical, her mention of a fast made me uneasy once again. I imagined some skinny, half-naked hermit sitting on a mountaintop, eating only nuts and wild berries (and garlic) while contemplating his navel. Once again, I thought, hey, maybe this really isn't for me. But I was determined to hear her out. I didn't have much to lose and maybe—just maybe— everything to gain. As skeptical as I was, as hard as I was trying NOT to believe her, all of this was beginning to make some sense.

"The fast will include apples and water for three days." Later, and over the following years, my investigation and experience would teach me the real value of the old Ben Franklin saying: "An apple a day keeps the doctor away." As with many old folk remedies, the medicinal benefits of fruit, and specifically of apples, have been recognized by healers and doctors for ages.

According to Dr. Alan Greene, health authority, there are at least five good reasons to eat "an apple a day":

- **Your Diet**-Apples are the perfect, portable snack, great tasting, energy-boosting, and free of fat.

- **Your Heart**-Research confirms it! The antioxidants found in apples help fight the damaging effects of LDL (bad cholesterol).

- **Your Lungs**-An apple a day strengthens lung function and can lower the incidence of lung cancer, as well.

- **Your Bones**-Apples contain the essential trace element, boron, which has been shown to strengthen bones-a good defense against osteoporosis.

- **Your Digestion**-Just one apple provides as much dietary fiber as a serving of bran cereal. (That's about one-fifth of the recommended daily intake of fiber.)

(2003)

Apples have also been shown to improve the mental abilities of people with Alzheimer's disease, Parkinson's disease, and other conditions associated with aging. A study done by food scientist Chang Y. Lee has shown that cancer cells in rats are actually killed by ingredients found in apples. (Aaronson 2004).

Of particular importance in the fast that I was to follow is the ingredient pectin, which is a gel-like substance, found just beneath the skin and in the core of many fruits, particularly the apple (*Columbia Encyclopedia 2005*).

Mary explained the value of apple pectin in this fast: "As the apples move through the bowel and the blood passes by the large intestine to deposit waste, the apple pectin will absorb it.

"The built up areas that have been re-poisoning the blood will break loose and leave. The lower bowel was not meant to put toxins back in the blood that way, as there is a barrier for that naturally in your body. Those built up areas, however, breech the barrier, and then," she explained, "you have all the toxins from the rotting waste and Candida going right back in."

I swallowed hard. "Ok," I said, not sure what else to say. This was all news to me but sounded reasonable. Somehow, I knew she had to be right.

Then, she went on to again tell me that the "acne" was really a symptom of a larger problem. It had nothing to do with genetics or too much oil.

"The body doesn't produce more of anything than it needs, oil or otherwise, unless it is ill. The body knows what it is doing!

Over time, I would come to share her appreciation for the body, especially for that marvelous human organ, the skin.

Constantly replenishing itself, the skin covers a whopping [20] square feet and constitutes 15 percent of our total body weight. In the three layers of one square inch of skin you'd find:

- 19 yards of blood vessels
- 65 hairs
- 78 yards of nerves
- 100 sebaceous glands
- 650 sweat glands
- 1,300 nerve endings
- 20,000 sensory cells
- 129,040 pores
- 9,500,000 cells

(Rodan and Fields 2004)

Mary continued: "I bet your dermatologists prescribed drying agents and creams."

"Yes," I said, "they did."

"I hear it all the time. All those do is dry out the skin so now you have dead skin cells blocking the pores compounding the problem. Your body is working hard to eliminate some of the waste and toxins through your skin and here it is all blocked." She sighed.

She continued by saying that I would need to follow a three-day cleansing fast and told me that it had been given in the 1940s for many ailments other than acne with fantastic results.
When people who incidentally had acne used it for other ailments, the acne disappeared.

As Dr. Joseph Rodrigo, M.D., has stated, "[The] intestinal track is [not only] the origin of disease, . . . it is also the origin of …healing." Dr. Rodrigo goes on to say, "I cannot emphasize enough how important the cleansing of [the] digestive system is to [the] health [of the human body]" (2005).

Probably no other aspect of my recovery from acne has been quite as interesting and life-changing as fasting. Evart Loomis, M.D., a noted expert on fasting sums it up this way:

Fasting is the world's most ancient and natural healing mechanism. Fasting triggers a truly wondrous cleansing process that reaches right down to each and every cell and tissue in the body. Within 24 hours of curtailing food intake, enzymes stop entering the stomach and travel instead into the intestines and into the bloodstream, where they circulate and gobble up all sorts of waste matter, including dead and damaged cells, unwelcome microbes, metabolic wastes, and pollutants [including heavy metals].

All organs and glands get a much-needed and well-deserved rest, during which their tissues are purified and rejuvenated and their functions balanced and regulated. . . . [T]he fast is an inward process and cannot be entered upon only from an outer approach with any expectation of a lasting benefit. The person must invariably be involved with the overall results. This therapeutic encounter is in direct contrast to the usual non-involvement in the physician-directed, disease-oriented medical practice of today (2005).

The historical background of the fast is extraordinary. For at least 10,000 years, fasting has been used in one way or another to rid mankind of suffering. Originally, perhaps, the suffering was of a spiritual, rather than physical, kind.

Fasting, which has been practiced for as long as history has been recorded, originally involved—and in some cultures and rituals still does involve—the limitation or suspension from food as well as other human activity including work, exercise, and sex. It has been a part of the religious ceremonies of practically all of the world's major religions.

Fasts were a common practice during the springtime and autumn, a kind of 'house-cleaning" for the body and the soul. Symbolically, fasting was used to place an individual in a state similar to death or birth. It was also a way to pay for one's sins, to clean one's soul, and to show one's sorrow for having offended a higher power.

Fasting is still practiced by people of many religions:

Fasting is practiced to this day amongst Roman Catholic, Orthodox Catholics, Jews and several Protestant sects, notably Episcopalians and Lutherans, as well as Muslims, Tibetan Buddhists and American Indians. The early Christian church saw fasting as . . . a voluntary method to prepare to receive Holy Communion and baptism. Christ is said to have fasted voluntarily alone in the desert east of Jerusalem for a full forty days and forty nights, at the end of which he encountered the temptations of Satan. (Kennedy 2005)

Sadly, as Ron Kennedy points out, it is probably the religious association with fasting [that] makes it difficult for us to access the value of fasting, living as we do in a generally anti-religious, anti-spiritual society devoted to the promise of science ultimately to deliver understanding of all things (2005).

Fasting has taken on a number of different objectives. For instance, in modern times, the hunger strike, a form of fasting, has been [used] as a political weapon. [P]olitical prisoners in various parts of the world, including conscientious objectors in the United States, have [used] hunger strikes [in protest against wars]. Mohandas Gandhi, leader of the struggle for India's freedom, undertook fasts occasionally to compel his followers to obey his precept of nonviolence. ("Fasting," Microsoft Encarta 98)

The fast was also used by Gandhi to highlight his cause for Indian independence before the world community. Just exactly when the fast became a common treatment for human physical ailments is not known. Presumably, early cultures noticed that when people participated in spiritual fasts certain chronic ailments responded favorably to the practice.

Also it is important to remember that early and more so-called "primitive" people did not make the distinction between mind, spirit, and body that "advanced" people of the twentieth and twenty-first century do. Holistic medicine was really holistic living for them.

As I was to discover in my research, fasting has proven to be an important and healthy habit in many societies, both new and old. "In modern Europe, reputable clinics that support therapeutic fasting are quite common. In Sweden it's practically a national sport" (Brown 2005).

Ron Kennedy probably best sums up the importance of fasting—and perhaps of holistic living in general—when he says:

Unless we take a smug, modern, pseudo-scientific point of view that the ancients were simply too stupid to know better than to fast, we are forced to ask ourselves what is in fasting which is so good as to deserve all this attention. Modern medicine does take this smug, modern, pseudo-scientific point of view and has bastardized the fast into its cousin, the diet, a technique for losing weight. [Interesting enough], losing weight and keeping it off is one of the few things which the ancients never claimed for the fast . . . . (2005)

Mary listed books for me to read and doctors who had verified the results. She told me, "Do your own research, and you will see. It's important for you to really know that you're on the right path to a cure. Your mind gets it, but you need to know it inside."

Mary smiled and her glasses slipped down even further. "Good grief!" I looked at my watch. "It's been two and a half hours," I said getting up to leave.

"I know!" she got up and unlocked the door. I hadn't even realized she had ever locked and closed it. I thanked her and left. As I got into my car, I wondered what she meant. "Know it inside?" Oh well, just her personality, I thought.

As I drove home, flashes of lightning danced across the sky making it purple.

"Good," I thought, maybe it will cool off to 90 degrees.

Acne Free For 18 Years

I have been acne-free for over 18 years. My visit that day with Mary started it. I did as she said, and I did my research. She was completely correct!

I read about various forms of the all-fruit fasts (like apples and grapes), including one version of an apple fast for many ailments from the 1940s by Edgar Cayce. Cayce (pronounced "KC") is considered by many to be the father of holistic medicine in America. "Decades ago, he was emphasizing the importance of attitudes, emotions, exercise, and the patient's role–physically, mentally, and spiritually–in the treatment of illness" (quoted at EdgarCayce.org). Cayce's recognition of the importance of diet foresaw the direction of health care. I read several doctors' works on the subject of all-fruit fasts, and they actually confirmed the results.

For many skin conditions, the fruit diet was a recommended step. In my research, I have also found that there are several "contributing factors" to acne.

Diet alone did not cure me; neither did all the antibiotics and drugs my dermatologists offered. Yet, I still conquered it. I found, over the years through working with other people, that there are three factors that contribute to acne:

1. Poor elimination of waste from the bowel (primary).

You see, the foods we eat today tend to be very high in sugar content and starches, like flour. Add these to the amount of unhealthy oils, and the colon can easily become packed with waste that should have been removed from the body but just sits there feeding bacteria back into the blood stream.

This leads to many illnesses, not just acne. So the poorly eliminating colon becomes a feeder of toxins the other organs must deal with. The liver becomes overtaxed. When it can no longer handle the large amounts of toxins, the skin, and other organs of the body, must pick up the slack in eliminating waste. Your body, if you remember, strives to maintain a balanced, healthy environment. Because the toxins are foreign to this environment, the body "knows" to expel them—anyway it can.

2. Dry built-up skin blocking the pores from over drying products.

Drying agents and over-the-counter products didn't do the trick, either. In fact, they often made it worse and more painful because of the build up of dry skin blocking even more pores. Here is why. Almost all of the drying agents, such as benzyl peroxide and salicylic acid, dry out the upper layers of the dermis (skin) and cause it to flake and peel.

Salicylic acid is the key additive in many skin-care products used to treat acne, calluses, dandruff, psoriasis, corns, and warts. Like benzyl peroxide, it causes affected skin cells to flake off.

However, as these agents dry the skin–the job they were designed to do–the flakes can build up and actually block pores where oil and bacteria can create infections and pustules. This can lead to deep inflammation and cystic acne breakouts— exactly the opposite effect of what you are trying to accomplish.

Cystic acne can be a very serious problem. Essentially, this kind of acne is defined as the occurrence of abscesses (localized infections) that are resistant to healing. Characteristics include:

- deep infections with large nodules or cysts
- infections that do not "come to a head" at the surface
- little or no discharge
- blackheads and whiteheads that may or may not be present
- very slowly healing infections that can become a chronic problem
- probable scarring.

3. Overgrowth of Candida Albicans yeast that puts toxins in the body and blood stream.

There has been much written on the condition of Candida infection. The compacted waste in the colon I spoke of contributes to the higher than normal presence of Candida yeast, which produces toxins of its own. These toxins add to the already heavy burden of the body trying to remove them. Almost every time Candida is brought under control, acne diminishes or disappears completely.

So drying agents and over-the-counter products didn't do the trick, either. In fact, they often made it worse and more painful because of the build up of dry skin blocking even more pores. Instead, I turned to alternative ways of dealing with my acne.

I tried the health food stores and even herbal treatments. I learned that some worked very well for others and saw some results on myself. For me, however, it was when I went outside of the usual course of acne treatment that I began to unravel the mystery of *why* I was having acne.

Now I had in front of me a new way to combat my acne, an inexpensive and very effective way to finally banish my acne. I have been acne free for eighteen years! The cleansing fast will be the primary method I will be recommending to you.

While reading up on herbal treatments for my acne as well as psychological and spiritual aspects of the condition and the negative feelings it creates, I was finally reading something that made sense to me! I read about acne being a result of the body trying to rid itself of toxins and how those of us with a genetic predisposition for oily skin and slow metabolisms usually have the worst symptoms.

You can't do much about having a genetic predisposition for something, such as oily skin. Certainly, oily skin had advantages for your ancestors. If, for example, your ancestors were from the sunny Mediterranean, oily skin probably kept them from sunburning and getting skin cancer. The same is true if you have ancestors from regions of the world with monsoon-like seasons. During frequent and torrential rainy seasons, essential body oils are easily washed away. None of this is your fault, of course, so blame your parents!

On the up side, …there are some advantages to having an oily hide, not the least of which becomes apparent with the steady passing of time. [O]ily skin tends to age better and wrinkle less than dry or normal skin. Today's curses; tomorrow's blessing. (Donsky et al)

Thank your parents too!

Teenagers have acne much more often than adults do, although the number of people with recurring outbreaks in adulthood is also increasing. No doubt the growing practice among American adults and children of eating poorly and exercising very little has led to colon problems and the retention and re-absorption of toxins by the body (autointoxication).

I read how you can detoxify the body and clear the reactions that cause the acne in the first place, just as Mary had said. This made sense to me, and I wondered what my practical licensed dermatologist would think about this approach.

There were also additional methods to cure even the most resistant acne with a little more time and effort. So I began the three-day fast. It was a simple, cleansing diet.

In order to detoxify the body completely, you needed to remove the metals and toxins in the liver that create acne breakouts.

A toxin can be defined as any substance that is harmful or irritating to the body. The number of toxins our body must neutralize or eliminate has increased dramatically during the twentieth and twenty-first centuries. We drink chemically treated water, breathe in more chemicals from factories and automobiles, and eat more processed foods. Toxins in our foods can result from additives that preserve either the appearance, shelf-life, or taste of what we eat. Pesticides, too, are a major source of toxins in our body. All medications have the potential to poison our bodies if they are taken in amounts large enough and over a period of time long enough.

These toxins become a problem to our health when the body fails to reduce or eliminate toxicity to a safe level. In our body, toxins are treated through the functions of several organs including 1) the liver, 2) the kidneys, 3) the intestines, and 4) the skin.

Of these, the liver, the largest gland in our body, is the chief organ of detoxification.

The blood draining the stomach and small intestine is transported directly to the liver, exposing it to relatively high amounts of ingested drugs or toxins. The liver provides a protective effect by altering . . .toxins and thereby neutralizing and/or increasing the removal of these foreign substances from the body. (Toxicology-Info.com)

The liver specifically deals with five sources of bodily toxins from:

1. food, alcohol, and other drugs

2. environmental pollutants
3. internally produced toxins
4. nitrogen-containing waste
5. energy production.   (Sodhi)

Fasting is one very successful method for detoxifying the body. I read through the instructions for the fast very carefully, and I will outline the directions and my experience for you.

"Eat nothing but apples for three days, drink water only and 3oz of grape juice the last day."

You also needed to massage pure castor oil into your affected skin each night before retiring. This was to help keep the pores open.

Castor oil is another of those great natural products that mankind has been using for hundreds of years. The specific uses for castor oil, however, have changed greatly over the years.

While it was Cayce who brought castor oil. . . to fame in the 20th century, the oil has a long and varied history of use as a healing agent in folk medicine around the world. According to a research report in a recent issue of the *Journal of Naturopathic Medicine,* castor bean seeds, believed to be 4,000 years old, have been found in Egyptian tombs, and historical records reveal the medicinal use of castor oil in Egypt (for eye irritations), India, China (for induction of childbirth and expulsion of the placenta), Persia (for epilepsy), Africa, Greece, Rome, Southern Europe, and the Americas. In ancient Rome, the castor plant was known as "Palma Christi," which [means] the "hand of Christ." (Gabbay)

Cayce described at least thirty ailments that responded favorably to the topical application (applied to the skin) of castor oil.

You also needed to do a very thorough internal cleansing of the bowel via an enema you could administer yourself or through a colonic irrigation given by a practitioner.

Enemas are performed for a variety of reasons:
- to hydrate (put water into) the body's systems;
- to remove waste;
- to stimulate peristalsis (the natural rhythm of the intestines);
- to repair the nerves, muscles, glands, circulatory, and immune systems;
- to reposition the intestines.

(Shea)

Furthermore, many different groups of people benefit from the use of occasional enemas:
- athletes, to improve the efficiency of their metabolisms;
- individuals during a period of life-style change or as a preventive measure;
- individuals with digestive distress, such as irritable bowel syndrome or chronic constipation;
- sufferers of chronic pain;
- individuals with compromised immune systems;

- pre-op (before surgery) and post-op (after surgery) patients;
- fasters;
- individuals who are working on certain kinds of emotional stress that they feel are centered in the intestines.

(Shea)

(For those who are unfamiliar with the enema or colonic process, I have included a great website belonging to a certified colon therapist.)

You needed to continue to use the castor oil every night for as long as you felt you receive benefit from it. Easy and inexpensive—still, I was skeptical.

Again, I read how this treatment had worked for people since the 1940s and was so effective that many did the "Apple or Grape Fast" once or twice a year to keep their acne—among other ailments—clear, even though none of them had it return.

Apples and humans have a long and proud history together. As the American naturalist "Henry David Thoreau, wrote, 'It is remarkable how closely the history of the apple tree is connected with that of man'" (quoted in Vegetarians in Paradise).

Although no one knows for sure where the apple originated, clearly the ancient Romans were the first to cultivate the fruit for human consumption. It was not long after, apparently, that people began to realize that the apple was not just a tasty fruit but was also a beneficial and healthy food.

Apples are easy on the digestive system and contain acids that stop fermentation in the intestines. They are high in fiber, which makes them a good aid in the elimination of the bowels. They also contain pectin, which is beneficial to the growth of good bacteria in the intestines.

Furthermore, they contain the same kind of antioxidants found in garlic, which has proven to fight cancer-causing free-radicals in the body.

As I said earlier, these results have been confirmed by several medical doctors.

Since nothing else cured my acne, I decided to try it. What did I have to lose? I was twenty-five years old and about to end my relationship with acne permanently. Now I am helping thousands of people do the same.

Even for the individual with resistant acne—the kind that reacts but needs more work—this diet is the beginning of a wonderful healing process that attacks the problem at its source. This is not a temporary "fix."

How The Program Works

Being a regular person and rather skeptical of such a simple solution, I wondered how it could possibly work. The only requirement is that the apples must be Red Delicious or Golden (**red grapes can be substituted by those people allergic to apples**) since they have more pectin to absorb the toxins in your system as your body digests them.

*Apples are recommended—but red grapes may be substituted for the apples for the three-day period. Use apples or grapes but NOT both, followed by two tablespoons of regular olive oil at the end of the last day. This helps the digestive process re-start.

The medicinal benefits of the olive tree have been known since biblical times. Moses, it is said, relieved olive farmers from compulsory service in the army because olive oil was so important to health and diet of the Israelites. The tree is mentioned in the bible often and has become a symbol of peace, happiness, and victory (the winners in the Olympics were once crowned with olive leaves) (tuberose.com).

Throughout history, the olive grew in importance as a medicine for a number of serious illnesses. Ingredients in the olive have been used to lower blood pressure in animals, to treat patients with malaria and particularly successful at reducing fevers, and to relieve muscle spasms. In the 1960s, a Dutch scientist isolated a substance in olive oil that has powerful antibiotic effects. Since then, olive oil has also been shown successful at fighting a number of viruses including some associated with the common cold (tuberose.com).

The water helps this process along, as well as a small amount of grape juice and the olive oil on the last day ensures that the apples are moved through and out of your system. You may eat as many apples as you can on all three days.

This might be a good place to mention the vital properties of nature's most underrated and yet richest gift: water. We–humans and all living things–are water-dependent creatures. Water has an important role in the spiritual lives of most nationalities and religions.

[I]n ancient times, the spiritual essence of water evoked a sense of wonder, reminding people that they were threads in the divine web of life. Foremost in the great creation stories and traditions of nearly every culture is the recognition that water gave birth to humankind, it was seen as a divine, life-giving, **healing, cleansing, renewing** force (emphasis added). (Epstein)

As historian Cathy Gutierrez explains: "The first mention of water for Judaism, and later Christianity, is found the first verse of Genesis: (Gutierrez)

In the beginning, God created the heavens and the earth. The earth was without form and void, and darkness was upon the face of the deep; and the Spirit of God was moving over the face of the waters. (Gen. 1:1-2)

Because it is usually so abundant and so readily available for Americans in the twenty-first century, most of us don't think of water often.

However, our ancestors and people now living in places where water is scarce have been aware of the value of good clean water. As Professor Mike Richards, an expert in the historical link between man and water, points out, "Beginning with the Industrial Revolution, . . . water increasingly became a hidden factor in human history. For many [Europeans and Americans, water] quite literally went underground, hidden from sight until one turned on a faucet or flushed a toilet."

(Richards)

What follows are some facts about water that perhaps you did not know.

- The human body is two-thirds water. That means if you are a man weighing 175 pounds, about 118 of those pounds are water; a 130-pound woman has about 87 pounds of water in her body.
- Although you can live up to several weeks without food (depending on your size), you will live less than a week without water.
- Water in the body must be constantly replenished. Even those of us who have minimal activity lose about 30 ounces of water a day through breathing, sweating, and the bowels.
- Our blood is about 80 percent water
- Muscles are about 75 percent water. (Men, therefore, have more water in their bodies than

women since men have more muscle mass. Fat, alas, has no water content!)

In the body, water has two critical jobs:

1. It carriers oxygen and food <u>to</u> every cell in the body; and
2. It removes toxins and wastes <u>from</u> every cell in the body.

Consequently, our bodies are in a constant state of balancing the intake and output of water. As we have seen before, the body's need for balance is always critical to its good health.

In short, water has about the same function in the human body as it does in nature in general. It keeps the "environment" clean and oxygenated (filled with oxygen). In addition, water in the human body has these secondary functions:

*   Keeps body temperature constant
*   Keeps joints lubricated so they can move easily
*   Keeps all organs of the body cushioned. Newborns are almost three-quarters water. "'That's mostly for cushioning,' says Felicia Busch, a spokesperson for the American Dietetic Association and specialist on the nutritional effects of water. 'Because of the birth process, they need a lot of cushioning.'" (Quoted in Mansfield)

The best way to replenish our water is by drinking it. You should not, however, wait until you are thirsty to drink water. Thirst is a sign of dehydration, a sign that the body is not getting enough water. It is almost impossible to drink too much water, so drinking it throughout the day is a good idea. Fortunately, most of the food we eat also has water in it.

A potato, for instance, is 80% water. Be careful of some foods and drinks, however. Coffee, colas, and alcohol actually act as diuretics, draining the body of its precious moisture, and should not be consumed often, if at all.

The program I am offering also requires an "internal cleansing" via enema or mild laxative to wash out the lower bowel on the second and third days. It is important NOT to reabsorb the very toxins you are working to remove.

For those unfamiliar with an enema, it is used in place of laxatives (which you should try not use) to make sure your colon is empty each day during the process. A mile laxative such as "Fletchers Castoria for Children" is ok if you just cannot do the water enema—**but I cannot guarantee the results without the enema**.

Let me take a moment here to talk about how the enema affects the body and what it will do for you. As I said before, waste matter builds up in the colon and is particularly a problem for people with high amounts of candida yeast in their systems. Sugars and starches lead to constipation and build up of this matter, and the colon becomes compacted with stretches of hard waste.

109

Just like corrosion inside a water pipe, the colon has a hard time moving waste out correctly, and the problem continues to get worse. The warm water enema used as directed will, over the course of the three days, soften, loosen, and remove these patches of incrusted fecal matter. In conjunction with the detoxifying effects of the apple fast, there just is no better way to correct and heal the colon.

The water, salt, and baking soda solution are highly effective for this reason. Enemas are perfectly safe and health building. They should <u>not</u> be used ongoing, day after day. Your body can become dependent on enemas like over-the-counter laxatives rather than its own mechanism—which is what we want—a healthy, regular colon. If you feel you must use the over the counter mixture, I cannot guarantee results.

Still, I have had some reports back that the Fletcher's Castoria has worked. You can also try one of the alternative methods, but again the apple fast is the number one method I recommend.

Fleet brand makes inexpensive enemas that come with simple instructions to follow—very easy and effective. I have also included extensive instructions for this procedure. This may sound a little unpleasant, but it truly isn't.

If a colonic irrigation service is available in your area, I would suggest that—where someone will administer it. An enema is simply the insertion of water into the lower bowl to wash out impacted debris and bacteria. On a

detox regimen such as the apple diet, this step is
imperative.

You need to make sure you are divesting yourself of the
apple fiber you've digested which has absorbed all the
toxins. In other words, you need to ensure you use the
restroom each day while on the diet. (Back to the enema
and how I was instructed to do the fast.)

I was thinking, "OK, apples, water, and enema…I can deal
with this for three days, no big deal."

So, I went to the store and bought about 30 apples, the
Fleet enemas, some Welch's grape juice, and olive oil. I
thought about the water, and decided to use bottled just to
be sure I was drinking the purest water possible.

With my apples, grape juice, olive oil, fleet enemas, and
bottled water, I spent far less than any prescription drug or
even over-the-counter product.

I went home and started to follow the plan. Three days
suddenly seemed very long; but then again, not so long
compared to the years of dealing with this embarrassing
skin condition.

The Steps for the Apple Fast Method

What you will need:

1) 10 or more Red Delicious Apples PER DAY!
Peel them before you eat them since most apple skins commercially produced have been sprayed with pesticides. (Jonathan will work as well.)

2) 3 Fleet enemas or whatever brand is available or an enema bag.

The enema bag will also work if you have one. With this you will need salt and baking soda. One teaspoon each in 1 quart of warm, NOT HOT water.

3) Plenty of water to drink.

Please have as much bottled or filtered tap water available. This way, you make sure you have it when you need to drink. The MORE water the BETTER! I drank 6-8 16 oz. bottles of water per day.

4) 3oz (juice glass) Welch's Grape Juice for the last day ONLY!

5) 2 tablespoons of olive oil on the last day ALSO!

113

Note: We get many requests from our clients for the products I recommend in this book including items you will want to use to maintain your results. For your convenience, the items can be found on our website address below. We are happy to offer them at below retail pricing and in the amounts needed to perform all the methods I used to end my acne battles forever.

http://www.acnefreein3days.com/easystartkit.html

Fasting is an age-old way to heal the body. It has been a form of healing throughout recorded history. It is even used by medical doctors of today for certain illnesses. Determining food allergies in a person is a good example: all food is stopped, and one food is reintroduced at a time to an individual until the culprit is discovered.

There are many different types of fasts. Some are one day, others three to seven days. Some fasts, such as religious-based fasts, may last months. Some fasts are complete fasts where only water is taken and no food what so ever. Some, such as the apple fast, are specialty fasts that are used to treat certain conditions in the body with a particular herb or food taken alone.

A fast works in the following way: by not eating food, the body completely expels all wastes and shuts down the digestive processes. This occurs in the 24-48 hour timeframe. The body begins digesting the oldest cells and fats that are stored.

As this occurs, the individual on the fast sometimes feels tired or has a headache as toxins and diseased tissues are digested at the cellular level.

This process occurs during days two and three of the fast. These symptoms are natural and usually pass. If you experience these discomforts, I suggest a cup of hot tea is fine; green tea is especially good. An old Chinese proverb says it best: "Better to be deprived of food for three days, than tea for one" ("The Miracle of Green Tea").

Although the Chinese have known the benefits of green tea for more than 4,000 years, American and European cultures have begun to appreciate it only recently.

Of the three kinds of tea–oolong, black, and green–green tea is the most healthy and beneficial. All three types of tea come from the same plant; the unfermented leaves of green tea are, however, the least processed, a fact shown in natural green color that is retained in this kind of tea.

This unfermented tea seems to provide a number of naturally healthy benefits and may be useful in the fight against the following:

- arthritis
- high cholesterol levels
- cardiovascular disease
- infections
- impaired immune function
- headaches
- depression

115

- viruses
- aging
- high blood sugar levels
- obesity

Green tea contains an antioxidant, EGCG, that is "at least 100 more times effective than vitamin C and 25 times more effective than vitamin E at protecting cells. . . from damage believed to be linked to cancer, heart disease, and other serious illnesses" (JapaneseGreenTeaOnline.com)

The introduction of the apples creates an accelerated detox process, and the apple pectin absorbs metals and toxins as it moves through the body. This is why it is imperative you follow the directions exactly—fasting works and it will help you to heal your acne condition.

Day 1: THIS DIET MUST BE FOLLOWED FOR THREE FULL 24-HOUR DAYS!

<u>Peel</u> and eat as many apples as you want and have as much water as you wish. I usually eat nine or ten apples; you can eat more, **depending on the level of your hunger.**

However, you MUST drink at least 60 ounces of water each day! You must use the castor oil on your skin! The <u>enema must be administered</u> at the end of the day.

<u>Instructions for a thorough lower bowel cleansing</u>. If you are on the apple fast, I cannot emphasize this step enough. An enema is simply the cleansing of the lower bowel with water – or water and salt or baking soda.

The reason this step is so important on this fast is that as the apples move through the digestive tract, they actually absorb toxins from the blood passing through from the liver.

If you do not ensure you have passed all the apples at the end of each day, you are going to reabsorb the toxins and not have very good results. Again, in some cities there are clinics available that do this. They give what are called "colonics."

Many of my clients in the UK and USA do this with fantastic results. However, you can achieve satisfactory results at home.

You will need to use mildly warm water (not hot water) to do the cleansing. If you are going to administer the enema to yourself, you will need to do the following.

1. Lying on your left side, insert enema tube per instructions on the box. If you are using a fleet pre-prepared enema, you will need to sit the bottle in hot water for three minutes to warm it. Vaseline can be used to make insertion easier.

Fleet store-bought enemas already have sodium in them. If your using an enema bag (also known as a douche apparatus), you will need to mix one quart of very mild to almost cool water with one teaspoon of salt and baking soda.

2. After inserting the tube, fill the lower bowel with water (empty the entire fleet enema, and if using the enema bag take in one half of the water in the bag.) Do this very slowly and maintain comfort. Hold for three to five minutes or until you have the urge to expel it.

After you expel it, do the same thing lying on the right side and then again in the "knee and chest to floor" bowing position. You will have rinsed out the lower bowel three times. You will need to reuse only one Fleet enema bottle per day since it is only good for one rinsing. Simply refill the bottle with warm water for positions two and three. It is important to do this every day of the fast and even again at the end of the first day "after" you finish the fast.

Please note—an enema performed correctly is completely safe and very effective. IF you would rather have it professionally done, please contact a clinic that performs the colonic. Most people fare just fine doing this part of the process themselves.

What to expect: I usually have no issues the first day. It's surprising how filling the apples can be. The castor oil will be thick but be sure to apply it every single evening.

Day 2:

<u>Peel</u> and eat five or six apples, more is fine, and drink plenty of water. Absolutely NO cheating with other foods. I find Day 2 to be the hardest to resist eating other foods.

You may have a few cramps and can do the enema anytime that day to relieve them. Just make sure you have the enema by the end of the day. Continue with the castor oil at night. Administer an enema at the end of the day.

What to expect: By the end of day 2, you could notice your acne calming down a little. I had no new sores appearing, and the cystic bumps calmed some. I felt "lighter" as well.

Some folks actually see their acne "act up" a little more the second and third day. **This is normal!** It means you are affecting your acne and is reflective of your system reacting.

Most of you will not see it get worse, but it will get better!

Day 3:

Eat the rest of your apples and drink plenty of water. At dinner, have a treat by drinking some grape juice! Continue with the castor oil, as the effects are cumulative. Take two tablespoons of olive oil to restart your digestive system.

Drink a full glass of grape juice around dinnertime, and have more than one if you wish. Have the enema again, at the end of the day.

What to expect: Day 3 should be the interesting day. You may notice that you're using the bathroom a little more than on the previous days.

You might also have a slight headache—much like a hangover. A hot shower will help with this. Drinking the green tea will also help this. You must drink lots of water! Drink at least 60 ounces.

You will notice the acne really calming down and much of the sores and bumps quickly receding. It is important to also continue with your water and grape juice.

Now, some folks see a slight improvement that continues every day for a month or so. For 98% of you, your acne will have cleared up in three days. For those with resistant acne that hangs on a little, you will need to read and do the methods for resistant acne. You have an extra step or two—BUT ALL acne sufferers would do well to read that section and follow the suggestions.

<u>Please note:</u> On the very rare occasions when I have had a report that the diet has not had as much effect as described, I always discover that either other food was taken, or the enema internal cleansing was skipped, or smoking or the use of drugs has occurred.

Since this has also been the case verified by the medical doctors I have referenced, I cannot be responsible for poor results as I leave the process of following directions up to you, the individual. Happily, it is rarely an issue.

The Result:

After three full days of following these very specific directions, I was pleasantly surprised to find that my skin looked very clear!

In fact, my acne completely DISAPPEARED on the fourth day! I also felt great, not to mention the five pounds I shed in the process!

After the First Three Days:

It is important to start with solid foods *slowly*. You can start with some soup and crackers, and a few hours later, if you feel good, you can have more.   I usually do not have a regular meal until Day 5. In other words, when the diet is over, don't jump in your car and run to McDonalds!

Maintaining the Results

The apples are the key. They cleansed the toxins, created better all-around health, and cured me of my acne. I find that eating as little sugar as possible helps maintain these benefits. You can even repeat the fast a couple of times per year to maintain overall health and wellness in addition to your clear skin. The fast should never be done more than once per month.

As I said, my acne has never returned. I realize, however, that there are those who just will not do the apple fast. It is the primary method I recommend.

Keep in mind, if you go back to old habits without continuing to take steps to balance the body, you will have the acne return. The body is going to do its job in removing toxins and waste.

There are other additional methods you can use in conjunction with the apple fast or alone. All have proven benefits. Only the apple fast, however, usually gives the three to four days result. It's easy, inexpensive, and highly effective. I maintain the results I have by drinking plenty of water.

I also strongly recommend taking odorless garlic supplements, vitamin C and acidophilus everyday. This along with the external use of castor oil as a steaming moisturizer and tea tree oil for fast healing of the occasional bump or blocked pore are what I have done to successfully keep acne away.

Although the full range of benefits provided by vitamin C is still being decided, the fact that it is essential to human life is certain. Strangely enough, humans are among the few living organisms, both animals and plants, that cannot produce ascorbic acid (vitamin C) themselves. Linus Pauling, a noted Nobel scientist, believed that "the failure to produce the chemical by an animal species is a genetic defect" shared by all humans (Pauling 1986).

Because the vitamin is water soluble–it dissolves in water and, therefore, is continuously flushed out of the body rather than being stored–it must be consumed regularly. Fortunately, many of the foods humans normally eat contain vitamin C.

These additional steps I recommend, along with eliminating sugar, virtually assure you of keeping acne a distant memory. Do you remember my talk about "paying the price"? Well, that is the small price you will pay for clear skin.

Please note that we get many requests for the products I recommend in this book including items you will want to use for maintaining your results. For your convenience, the items can be found on our website at…

http://www.acnefreein3days.com/easystartkit.html

We are happy to offer them at below retail pricing and in the amounts needed to perform all the methods I used to end my acne battles forever.

Special Instructions for Reducing and Removing Facial Acne Scars

One of the unpleasant ramifications of acne is the resulting scarring that can occur. Scarring is particularly the case where you have cystic acne as I did.

Once the acne is cleared, it often leaves behind pockmarks, red broken veins, and even deep thickened skin in the form of impressions. These small indentations cause an uneven reflection of light and so the marks look darker and worse than they really are.

Make-up is of little use because the skin is still uneven and impressions under the make-up are still visible. After my acne was cleared, I became determined to get the scars removed. "Skin resurfacing" is an expensive undertaking if you go the medical routes of laser surgery, dermabraision treatments, or the oxalate crystals treatments.

None of these alternatives are guaranteed and can cause even more skin damage. My choice was to look at the acid peels, but they, too, were quite pricey and could have complications.

The depth of the scarring (wrinkle, fine lines, pigment, or severe scar) determines the depth of the peeling necessary.

With an intermediate or deep peel, additional scarring, infection, skin darkening, and skin lightening may occur. Patients with darker skin pigmentation are especially poor candidates for a deep skin peel.

However, I did find a company that carries an extremely effective product called "Skin Peel 4000." It was reasonable in price and had four levels of peels, depending on how deep you needed to have your skin peeled.

The peels had no harsh chemicals and no complications. I was very impressed with their level of service as well. I did the peel and my scarring was dramatically reduced, by at least 90%.

I get compliments on my skin—something I could only dream about in the past. I tried the peels, and to my amazement, they worked extremely well.

You see my picture and the results I have had. Skin Peel 4000 is produced by a respected company called Skin Culture. Their website is…

http://www.skincultureusa.com

Resistant Acne Methods

A few of you may have very resistant acne. If you have completed the apple fast according to instructions and still have a lot of sores, you will want to continue with the alternative methods because the apple fast did work. Yes, I said the apple fast did work!

You may need to do the apple fast again a couple of times over a three-month period. Each time you will be removing more of what is causing your problems.

Once you have completely detoxed your body, your skin will follow. Or if you just don't think you can do the apple fast, then you will need to do the alternative methods.

For you it may take longer for the acne to "clear." Those methods work well *over time*. Everyone is different, and the results occur in different amounts of time.

All should give you results within a 90-day period. You can always contact me for additional advice and help— again, one of the great things about having direct access to me online.

Sometimes, even after the fast is over, you may feel your acne gets a little "worse" but DO NOT get discouraged. This is a GREAT sign because now you are seeing for yourself that your acne is *reactive* to what you are doing. You must stay the course!

Your acne is very likely caused by Candida albicans—or yeast. This is the same yeast that causes yeast infections in women and thrush (the white coating on your tongue when you're taking antibiotics).

I have spent a lot of time helping folks with this problem. You are going to have to eliminate sugar from your diet for a while – period. You are also going to have to take some garlic tablets (odorless), as this will help the dying off process with your acne and Candida.

A lot has been written about these types of yeast infections in men, women, and children. They affect your immune system greatly. Those of you with children will note that after a round of antibiotics is prescribed, your child often gets a case of thrush or an ear infection.

There are medications available to help cure over-populations of Candida in your system. I recommend this natural method.

Candida Yeast Infection
"Nutrition Method"

I also know that if you are regularly consuming a high concentration of processed-food, you may have to do two or three of these diets over a period of three to five months to get the greatest benefit.

The naturally occurring yeast Candida albicans in our bodies often increases our acne problems. It is one of the reasons you can have so many toxins in the body. I learned this personally.

This yeast can get out of control from the very antibiotics dermatologists prescribe! The antibiotics kill off the beneficial bacteria in your system, acidophilus, which must be present to keep the yeast down. How many times have antibiotics caused thrush and even yeast infections?

This is all verified by science—not me. So, by making a few dietary changes (removing sugar), you can reduce Candida albicans dramatically and help the apple fast to remain effective.

Remove as much sugar and refined foods as possible from your diet and supplement your acidophilus b with a pill form. These small changes will reap for you years of benefits.

Acidophilus can be found at any grocery store or drug store and is very inexpensive. If you have reactive and resistant acne, this will clear it up.

I have yet to meet one person who—after the diets and internal cleansing (followed correctly) and removing all sugar and taking acidophilus and garlic tablets—did not completely put their acne in remission and cure it.

This takes a little time and effort, but the results can absolutely amaze you. Candida causes problems by producing toxins that have to be eliminated from your body.

Everybody has some Candida albicans, but when it gets out of control, it causes problems like acne and yeast infections. When you take the antibiotics they kill every bacterium—beneficial and/or otherwise that keep the Candida under control.

For this reason, you need the acidophilus b—to replenish the good bacteria—and the odorless garlic—to kill the yeast. You WILL get rid of your acne by following these steps.

Again, it is not as speedy, but the apple diet has prepared your system for this important cleansing. Even if you did not do the apple diet, the beneficial results will occur over time.

Castor Oil/ HOT Steam Method for Opening the Pores of the Skin.

What you will need: Small bottle of castor oil (available at any drug or grocery/health food store), washcloth, and hot water. This procedure is very effective for facial acne and was recommended to me by a dermatologist, believe it or not!

It is great if used in conjunction with the apple fast but can be used alone.

Instructions:

Daily and ongoing—steam face with hot (not hot enough to burn) washcloth. You must do this for a **MINIMUM** of 20 minutes in the morning and 20 minutes at night.

Every evening after you complete the steam session, you will massage the castor oil into the skin. Usually about a half a teaspoon is enough.

Leave on overnight and wash off in the morning *before* your 20-minute steam session. Do this daily. Results are visible in one to two weeks.

Herbal Methods

I am often asked, do herbs really work for acne? Yes, from what I have seen, they do. The thing is they work slowly while building gradual results.

Most internally taken herbs like Tahebo flush the toxins out, so the body can dispose of them. The problem is that since the body is taking care of it, your acne is likely to get worse temporarily.

Most folks start the process and just give up before they see the results. I am going to list the herbs associated with clearing up acne. If you decide to use the herbal methods, you must follow the instructions that come with the herb.

Aloe Vera, Bistort, Burdock, Castor Oil, Cayenne, Chaparral, Chickweed, Chlorophyll, Dandelion, Echinacea, Ginseng, Red Clover, Redmond Clay, Sarsaparilla, Tahebo Tee, Tea Tree Oil, Valerian Root, White Oak Bark, Yellow Dock.

I recommend the Tahebo and Melaluca Oil (Tea Tree oil) externally.

133

Melaluca Oil (Tea Tree oil) was probably first used by Aborigines in Australia to treat infections of the feet. The Tea Tree is grown, in fact, only in Australia, which exports 700 million tons of it annually. It may help to…

- **treat cuts, scrapes, insect bites and stings, and other minor skin wounds and irritations:** Because the Tea Tree oil combines easily with body oils and lessens the possibility of infections and the likelihood of scarring;
- **Shorten the course of vaginal yeast infections (Candida albicans);**
- **Treat head lice;**
- **Gently control acne.**

Essential Oil Method

Additional methods for clearing acne use topical application of essential oils. Essential oils are oils like menthol, eucalyptus, and tea tree oil that have antiseptic properties.

Essential oils are often referred to as "fragrant oils," the oils that are in many plants and used in perfumes. Although the healing powers of essential oils have been known for thousands of years–the ancient Mesopotamians actually had a machine that pressed the essential oils from plants 5,000 years ago– Europeans did not use them until fairly recently in history. A French doctor in the 1920s used lavender oil to heal a severe burn on his own body.

Another French doctor used essential oils during World War II to treat soldiers.

Essential oils cannot be taken into the body by ingestion (swallowing). They enter the body in two ways: through the nose and through the skin. They are extremely concentrated; in fact, the oil made from roses requires 4,000 pounds of rose petals to make one pound of essential rose oil (obviously, it is also very expensive) (Dupler).

Scientists now believe the essential oils can kill bacteria, fungi, and parasites. Most everyone is familiar with Listerine mouthwash. It is well known for its ability to sterilize the mouth and actually kill germs (bacteria) in the mouth responsible for gingivitis and periodontal disease.

Listerine accomplishes this through its ingredients of essential oils. The only essential oil I recommend, with which I have seen results, is Melaleuca oil. It can be purchased in almost every country and even easily purchased online. It's an all-natural oil derived from a tree in Australia. It is very powerful and yields dramatic results. Health food stores carry it. Follow the same directions for the castor oil method substituting the Melaleuca oil for the castor oil.

Please note that we get many requests for the products I recommend in this book including items you will want to use for the resistance acne methods. For your convenience, the items can be found on our website at…

http://www.acnefreein3days.com/easystartkit.html

135

We are happy to offer them at below retail pricing and in the amounts needed to perform all the methods I used to end my acne battles forever.

Reactive Foods That Can Aggravate Acne

During my challenges with my acne and over the years, I have come to the conclusion that certain foods do, in fact, aggravate acne conditions. In the case of Candida infections that are causing acne, this is almost always true.

Not all foods react the same with all people. The exception is that sugar always feeds a Candida infection and should be cut out as completely as possible in these cases.

The following is a list of foods that aggravate acne and cause Candida reactions to occur. There will probably be some surprises in the list.

Foods known to increase breakouts and Candida reactions

Caffeine—sodas and chocolate. Caffeine is a stimulant and can be found in many different foods. Coffee and cola are the more well-know examples, but caffeine is also in many other foods. The stimulant properties in caffeine seem to aggravate both acne breakouts and Candida infections.

Sugars—particularly refined such as white and powdered. Sugar is also in many different foods. In its natural form, such as in fruit (fructose), it is easily digested and managed by the body.

In its highly concentrated and refined form, it wreaks havoc on the body, especially in people who are suffering with Candida infections. The Candida yeast in the body must have sugar to grow and thrive. Cutting all refined sugar, and even natural sugar for a time, is the best way to eliminate Candida yeast overgrowth.

When I was at the height of my battle with acne, I can remember watching as the bumps on my face became seriously inflamed before I could even finish my "Big Gulp" of Coca Cola from the local 7-11!

Vinegar—also in many foods, from canned veggies to catsup, mustard, and salad dressing. Vinegar doesn't cause problems for all individuals, but many have sensitivity to it and do not even know it.

MSG—monosodium glutamate is found in most processed foods. Many people have sensitivities to MSG and in some people who are highly allergic to it, MSG can even be deadly. MSG is required to be listed on all foods, as it is added as a flavor enhancer and preservative.

Some symptoms of MSG sensitivity are extreme tiredness and sleepiness right after ingesting it. Skin reactions usually occur within 24 hours.

Bananas—Believe it or not, a lot of people have high skin sensitivity to bananas. Usually, these same people have an acute sensitivity to pineapple as well.

138

Iodine—such as in seafood like shrimp and lobster. Most people with sensitivities to seafood already know they have a problem. What a lot of acne and Candida sufferers don't know is, even if they seem to be able to eat seafood with no trouble, the iodine content has been shown to aggravate acne breakouts. The iodine seems to release a lot of stored toxins in the blood and leads to greater and more prolonged breakouts.

Dark colas—The coloring used in colas and syrups are artificial and can also excite acne conditions. Dark cold drinks are notorious because they contain so much more of the additives that can harm the body.

Staying away from dark colas will usually help tame acne breakouts. If you're someone with acne and drinks a lot of dark cold drinks, then you should consider eliminating them or greatly reducing your consumption of them.

Hydrogenated oils—I have said many times that oils in and of themselves are very healthy for the body. According to extensive research, olive, peanut, and canola are the best oils available. However, some brands of oils, especially the vegetable oils, are often hydrogenated.

Hydrogenation is a process where heated hydrogen molecules are pumped through the oil to add shelf life. Many people are sensitive to this process. Studies have shown there are many health disadvantages from eating oils that have gone through this process.

Animal lard—Animal fats are much different in their nature than are vegetable fats. Animal lard is rancid.

Look at it this way, fat begins to decompose naturally just like tissue. This is a natural process of nature.

As it breaks down, it creates toxins, but vegetable fats do not undergo the same process. Any kind of animal lard is not good for the body and can really create a good environment for Candida infections to grow and prosper.

Tomatoes—Many people with acne are more sensitive to high amounts of acids found in tomatoes. Tomatoes are so good for you: I rarely recommend cutting them unless you discover your acne is worse after eating them.

The healthful benefits of tomatoes are so great they should be eaten almost every day. However, if you find the breakouts you experience get worse after eating tomatoes, then you should stop eating them for a while.

Once your acne is under control, you can look at adding them back to the diet in small portions, until you find the amount you can tolerate without problems.

White potatoes—White potatoes are starchy foods. Taken in high amounts, they can raise blood sugars and feed Candida infections. Red potatoes are the best choice for meal preparation.

Red potatoes do not raise blood sugar and are broken down into a high glucose food. In fact, they have much more fiber, which is good for everyone and especially those fighting Candida yeast infections.

White Flour—This is obviously not recommended! This processed food creates so much trouble for the colon and is the number one contributor to binding and poor eliminations.

Flour becomes a pasty, hard-to-digest item for the body. This high starch also feeds Candida, and when combined with sugar and fat, it becomes what I call the "triple threat." Interesting enough, it is the primary ingredient in many "Western" foods.

Alcohol—In any form, alcohol slows the metabolism and feeds Candida. On top of that, all beers have some form of yeast used in the processing stages, which makes it an item Candida sufferers must remove from their diets.

Yeast—While the yeast used in foods (a form of mold) is not in and of itself unhealthy, because of the sensitivity in the body to yeast in Candida-infected people, it creates reactions including breakouts. The body sees yeast as yeast, and doesn't see a difference between the fight against Candida yeast and the yeast in that piece of bread you are eating.

Smoked meats—Smoked meats and nuts usually contain MSG, which we have already covered. In addition, there are usually high amounts of artificial additives that many acne and Candida sufferers react to.

Smoked cheeses—(same as above) Best to avoid all smoked meats, cheeses, and nuts.

141

Wine—Same as alcohol, with the addition that the high concentration of tannins in the darker wines causes breakouts in many people.

Molded foods such as bleu cheese—Most people with Candida and acne are more sensitive to molds of any kind. I couldn't even tolerate going into a basement for even a minute for many years.

In fact, even though I am acne and Candida free now—a moldy house, car, or basement, often sends me into dizzy spells, sneezing, and a cramping sick feeling. Avoiding all molds—especially bleu cheeses.

Mushrooms (uncooked)—Mushrooms are relatives of yeast. Even though they are one of my favorite foods, they can cause problems for many people. Again, in some individuals the body has an allergic reaction to mushrooms that is just like yeast. If you have increased breakouts or do not feel well after eating mushrooms, simply cut them from your diet.

By looking at how your body individually reacts to the foods you eat, you can speed up the healing process. Just pay attention to when your breakouts occur or get worse, and track what you do and eat on those days and the day just before the breakout. You will see a connection to some of the foods you eat. Everyone is different so use this list as a guide—not a letter of law.

Frequently Asked Questions

Q. *Can I eat something, at least a snack, while on the apple fast?*

A. For the apple or grape fast to be effective, it needs to be followed as outlined—apples/grapes and water—period. You cannot eat or drink anything else.

Q. *Do I have to do the enema part, and do I have to do it three times each evening?*

A. You are really doing only ONE enema—with 3 parts. For the first part, you will be using the saline solution already provided in the enema bottle. For the second and third parts, you will be refilling the bottle with warm water.

Done as directed, it is the most effective way to cleanse the lower bowel. Following the directions is not harmful or uncomfortable in the least. Plus, you will be sticking to the fleet enema directions that clearly state you should only perform one enema in a 24-hour period.

Q. *I completed the fast, but I still have some breakouts or have seen no change in my skin.*

A. Some people, even the ones who follow the fast and enema process correctly as outlined, still have some breakout areas. This is due to a severe build up of waste in the lower bowel, and the fast may need to be repeated up to two more times over a three to four month period to get the complete effect. It is recommended that you wait three weeks between doing another three-day fast. In the meantime, you should begin using the Resistant Acne Methods as outlined. There can also be a problem with the Candida yeast in the system and the method for dealing with that is included in this book (Resistant Acne Methods).

If your acne appears to actually get a little worse, then you are having what is termed a "die-off" reaction to the Candida that is being killed by the healthy bacteria. Do not panic! This is temporary, and in a few days you should see substantial improvement as long as you stay the course.

Q. *What is the next step after completing the three-day fast?*

A. The next step is to follow the Resistant Acne Methods. The reasoning is provided in that particular section.

Q. *Will the apple fast remove scars?*

A. While the apple fast will not remove scars, it will *lighten* them. Over time, the redness will subside. For more information and products I recommend for scar removal, please visit Skin Cultures website, **http://www.skincultureusa.com**.

Q. *What kind of soap is good to use?*

A. I always recommend foaming facial cleansers like Olay and Neutrogena. They contain no soap, which is very drying to the skin. Soap also throws the skins PH balance off. Bath and Body stores carry excellent clear glycerin soaps that will cut facial oils without over drying.

Q. *Can I get results without using the apple fast?*

A. The apple fast is "the" tool to get internal cleansing done. However, success has been documented by following the other methods such as the one for combating Candida infections. Steaming with castor or essential oils and cutting out all sugary foods works wonders over time as well.

Q. *I am allergic to apples and grapes, what can I do?*

A. For those of you allergic to apples and grapes, I would recommend for you to start following the Resistant Acne Methods. Although they will not provide results in three days like the fast, they will provide similar lasting results in only a matter of weeks.

Q. *Is it safe to do the apple fast while pregnant or breastfeeding? If not, what can I do?*

A. If you are pregnant or breastfeeding, then you will not be able to perform the apple fast during that time period. The apple fast is safe for you to do, but it is not recommended because for some people it does deplete the amount of nutrients available for the body to process during the three days.

You do not want your child to miss out on those important nutrients. I would recommend for you to start following the Resistant Acne Methods. Once you are done with your

pregnancy or breastfeeding, then you can proceed with the apple fast.

Q. *I can't seem to find castor oil in my area. In fact, I am having a hard time finding all of the products you recommend. Where can I purchase them online?*

A. Follow through to the next link and you will be provided with the ability to purchase castor oil online. You can also purchase any of the other products recommended in the book.

http://www.acnefreein3days.com/easystartkit.html

If you have additional questions not covered here or in the book at large, we welcome an email from you. Please email us at **admin@acnefreein3days.com.

Final Thoughts

Getting rid of my acne has greatly enhanced my life. I learned that not all problems could be solved by "consensus reality solutions."

Drugs may help with the symptoms, but they have their own negative side effects and don't necessarily affect the origin of the problem. I personally try to maintain balance without them.

This has been my personal experience about the beneficial results I attained from my quest to learn about my own acne condition.

It is heartening to see that even doctors such as the famous Dr. Atkins speak at length about acne and Candida infections— even in his famous weight loss plan.

More and more of what I have shared with you is being recognized—recognized because it works!

Disclaimer: "I recommend that you always check with your doctor before changing your diet or health routine. Again, I do not treat or cure any disease. I am simply sharing my personal experience."

Glossary

Abscesses - A collection of pus or purulent matter in any tissue or organ of the body; localized infections

Accutane – (isotretinoin) controversial drug, chemically related to Vitamin A, that works against acne by stopping skin pores from producing sebum

Acidophilus b. (Lactobacillus acidophilus) - a type of "friendly" bacteria. Many yogurts contain acidophilus, but, unfortunately, yogurt usually contains some form of sugar or fruit, too

Acne - a pustular affection of the skin, due to changes in the sebaceous glands; an inflammatory disease involving the sebaceous glands of the skin

Acne Vulgaris - the most common form of acne; usually affects people from puberty to young adulthood

Acupuncture - (Chinese) treatment of pain or disease by inserting the tips of needles at specific points on the skin

Adolescence - the time period between the beginning of puberty and adulthood

Affliction - 1) a state of great suffering and distress due to adversity, 2) a condition of suffering or distress due to ill health, 3) a cause of great suffering and distress

149

Glossary

Allopathy - traditional, proven healthcare

Alternative Healthcare - (sometimes referred to as "holistic healthcare") is based on a philosophy that looks at the whole person and the relationship between the parts of the body and the whole body

Antibiotic - a chemical substance derivable from a mold or bacterium that kills micro organisms and cures infections

Autointoxication – (bowel toxemia), poisoning, or the state of being poisoned, from toxic substances produced within the body

Bacterium – (pl. Bacteria) single-celled or non cellular spherical or spiral or rod-shaped organisms lacking chlorophyll that reproduce by fission

Blackhead - a black-tipped plug clogging a pore of the skin

Blemish - any mark of deformity or injury, whether physical or moral; anything that diminishes beauty, or renders imperfect that which is otherwise well formed; that which impairs reputation

Bowel - the part of the alimentary canal between the stomach and the anus

Candida Albicans - the most common yeast found in the human body and the cause of most so-called yeast infections

150

Castor Oil - a mild cathartic oil, expressed or extracted from the seeds of the Palma Christi, a plant, Ricinus communis, with ornamental peltate and palmately cleft foliage, growing as a woody perennial in the tropics

Chemotherapy - the use of chemical agents to treat or control disease (or mental illness)

Collagen - The chemical basis of ordinary connective tissue, as of tendons or sinews and of bone

Colon - the part of the large intestine between the cecum and the rectum; it extracts moisture from food residues before they are excreted

Colonic Irrigation - irrigation of the colon for cleansing purposes by injecting large amounts of fluid high into the colon

Comedo – (pl. Comedone) a small nodule or cystic tumor, common on the nose, etc., which on pressure allows the escape of a yellow wormlike mass of retained oily secretion, with a black head

Constipation - difficult or infrequent bowel movements resulting from prolonged bowel transit times (the time it takes food to be digested and then eliminated from the body)

Cosmeceutical - a word formed from the words "cosmetics" and "pharmaceutical" products are those remedies "marketed as cosmetics that purportedly have biologically active ingredients that affect the user" (Tsao 2004)

Cyst - 1) a closed sac that develops abnormally in some body structure, 2) a small anatomically normal sac or bladder like structure (especially one containing fluid)

Cystic Acne – also called acne vulgaris

Dermabrasion - essentially a kind of sanding of the skin. Using a motorized burr, the doctor (usually a plastic surgeon) levels out the surrounding surface skin

Dermatologist - a doctor who specializes in the physiology and pathology of the skin

Dermis - the deep vascular inner layer of the skin

Detoxify - remove poison from

Echinacea - small genus of North American coarse perennial herbs, to boost the immune system and to relieve flu-like symptoms

Enema - injection of a liquid through the anus to stimulate evacuation

Evolutionary - of or relating to or produced by evolution

Exfoliation - the peeling off in flakes or scales of dead skin

Fasting - abstaining from food; to omit to take nourishment in whole or in part; to go hungry; a common treatment for human physical ailments

Follicle - a small cavity, tubular depression, or sac

Gastrointestinal Tract (GIT) - tubular passage of mucous membrane and muscle extending about 8.3 meters from mouth to anus; functions in digestion and elimination

Google – To search the Web using the Google search engine, http://www.google.com

Hair Follicle - a small tubular cavity containing the root of a hair

Halo Effect – According to Dr. Mona Phillips, who teaches sociology at Spellman College, the "halo effect" refers to the tendency to associate a cluster of positive characteristics with a positive physical appearance. "People assume that if someone is attractive, then they have [other] good qualities [as well" (quoted in Reyes 2001).

Holistic - emphasizing the organic or functional relation between parts and the whole

Hormone - A chemical substance formed in one organ and carried in the circulation to another organ on which it exerts a stimulating effect

Inflammation - a response of body tissues to injury or

153

irritation; characterized by pain and swelling and redness and heat

Keratin - A nitrogenous substance, or mixture of substances, containing sulphur in a loose state of combination, and forming the chemical basis of epidermal tissues, such as horn, hair, feathers, and the like

Laser Surgery - light amplification by stimulated emission of radiation; controlled burning of the affected area with intense light waves. Lasers are popular because they cause little if any bleeding. In fact, the laser "vaporizes superficial layers of facial skin

Lesion - any visible abnormal structural change in a bodily part

Melaleuca Oil - all-natural oil derived from a tree in Australia

Metabolism - series of chemical changes which take place in an organism, by means of which food is manufactured and utilized and waste materials are eliminated

Microflora - good bacteria that live naturally in our bodies

Nausea - any sickness of the stomach accompanied with a propensity to vomit

Nodule - a firm, severe lesion that extends into the deep layers of the skin

Papule - a small, solid bump on the skin

Pathogenic - able to cause disease; "infective agents"; "pathogenic bacteria"

Pectin - a gel-like substance found just beneath the skin and in the core of many fruits, particularly the apple

Pharmacology - the science or study of drugs: their preparation and properties and uses and effects

Phosphoric Acid - an acid used in fertilizers and soaps

Pore - One of the minute orifices in an animal or vegetable membrane, for transpiration, absorption, etc.

Propionibacterium Acnes (P. Acnes) - the most common gram-positive, non-spore forming, anaerobic rod encountered in clinical specimens; the bacterium usually responsible for acne infections; the causative agent of acne vulgaris (pimples)

Pus - the body's white blood cells that attack the plugged pore and fight infection

Pustule - a small inflamed elevation of skin containing pus

Psychic Trauma – an emotional wound or shock often having long-lasting effects

Remission - an abatement in intensity or degree (as in the manifestations of a disease)

St. John's Wort - any of numerous plants of the genus

Hypericum having yellow flowers and transparently dotted leaves, for the treatment of mild depression

Salicylic Acid - a white crystalline substance with a bitter aftertaste; used as a fungicide or in making aspirin or dyes or perfumes; the key additive in many skin-care products used to treat acne, callouses, dandruff, psoriasis, corns, and warts

Scarring - marks left by the healing of injured tissue

Sebum - the oily secretion of the sebaceous glands

Sociologist - a social scientist who studies the institutions and development of human society

Therapy - (medicine) the act of caring for someone

Thrush - candidiasis of the oral cavity; seen mostly in infants or debilitated adults

Toxin - poisonous product formed by pathogenic bacteria

Whitehead - a small whitish lump in the skin due to a clogged sebaceous gland

References

"Acne Myths." Skincarephysicians.com

Acne-Treatments-Guide.com

"Alternative Medicine: How Popular Is Alternative
Medicine?" holisticonline.com

"Antibiotics!" liferesearchuniversal.com

"Approaching Complementary and Alternative Therapies."
holisticonline.com

American Academy of Dermatology, quoted in Amanda
Gardner, "Acne Leaves Emotional Scars, Too," in
HealthDay at healthcentral.com

Baker, Mitzi. "Young Adults' Heath Habits Are Worse
Than Ten Years Ago, Researchers Say." *Stanford
Report*. news-service.stanford.edu (September 24,
2004).

Bremner, Douglas. "Give Me Accutane."
skincarehealthy.com

Brown, Lonny J. "Adventures in Therapeutic Fasting," in
Shirley's Wellness Café.com

157

Busch, Felicia. "What Percentage of the Human Body Is Water, and How Is This Determined?" *The Boston Globe Extra net.* Boston.com/globe

"Case for Strong Antibiotics Regulations, The," physics.ohio-state.edu

Cayce, Edgar. EdgarCayce.org

Clapp, Ken. "America's Bad Habits Are Bloating Health-Care Costs." In *The Columbus Dispatch* (March 14, 2005).

"Constipation." DigestivePlus.com

"Do Attractive People Get Better Treatment Than Others?" *JET* (September 3, 2001).

Donsky, Howard; Kenneth Nelder; Hilliard H. Pearlstein. *The Doctor's Book of Home Remedies.* Rodale Books.

Dupler, Douglas. "Essential Oils." *Gale Encyclopedia of Alternative Medicine,* Gale Group (2001).

EHC.com

Epstein, Nadine and Rosita Arvigo. "Spiritual Bathing," *Spirituality and Health Magazine* (July-August 2003).

"Fasting." *Microsoft Encarta*

Feldman, Stephen; Rachel E. Careccia; Kelly L. Barham; John Hancox. "Diagnosis and Treatment of Acne." findarticles.com (2004).

Fried, Richard, quoted in Amanda Gardner, "Acne Leaves Emotional Scars, Too," in *HealthDay* at healthcentral.com

Fryhofer, Sandra Adamson. acponline.org

Gabbay, Simone. "Castor Oil: Modern Uses for an Old Folk Remedy." Annieappleseedproject.org/castoroiluses.html

Greeley, Alexandra. "Cosmetic Laser Surgery," *FDA Consumer Magazine* (publication CFDA 00-4272). (May-June 2000, with revisions made in August 2000).

Greene, Alan. "An Apple a Day?" (October 24, 2003).

Grieve, Mrs. M. "Garlic." Botanical.com

Gutuerrez, Cathy. "Water in History," *The Mystery, Art, and Science of Water*. Chris Witcombe and Sang Hwang, Sweet Briar College.

Hawrelak, Jason A. and Stephen P. Myers. "The Case of Intestinal Dysbiosis: A Review," *Alternative Medicine Review* (June 2004).

"Herbal Medicine." Umn.edu/altmed

Horovitz, Bruce. *USA Today.* usatoday.com

JapaneseGreenTeaOnline.com

"Journey to Wellness." wabe.org

Kava, Ruth. "Unhealthy Lifestyle" (April 16, 2003).
    techcentralstation.com

Kennedy, Ron. "History of Fasting." medicallibrary.com

Lee, Chang Y. study cited in Lauren Aaronson,
    Psychology Today (December 10, 2004).

Levine, Beth. "Teen Torment: Acne Can Scar More Than
    Skin," in *The Stanford Advocate* (online partner of
    the *Winston-Salem Journal* (June 21, 2005).

Loftus, Jean. InfoPlasticSurgery.com

Loomis, Evart. Quoted in "Therapeutic Fasting," Shirley's
    Wellness Café 2005.

Maghaddam, Fathali M. "Beauty in Everyday Life."
    healthandage.com

Martino, Russell J. "Colas, Soft Drinks and Your Health."
    totalhealthdynamics.com/soft_drinks.htm

Merritt (first name not given) in *Occupational Outlook
    Handbook,* Bureau of Labor Statistics (March
    2001). Umsl.edu/services/govdocs

National Institute of Health Conferences (November 5, 1977). Mdanderson.org

Pauling, Linus. *How to Live Longer and Feel Better*, W.H. Freeman and Company (1986). en.wikipedia.org

Perkins, Stephen, quoted in Greeley.

"Miracle of Green Tea." Quoted by Rhonda Perkinson. chinesefood.about.com

Phillips, Mona, quoted in Karla Reyes, "Appearance Proves Important." boonebraves.ocps.net (2001).

Richards, Mike. "Water in History," *The Mystery, Art, and Science of Water*. Chris Witcombe and Sang Hwang, Sweet Briar College.

Rodan, Katie, and Kathy Fields. "Skin Under Siege," chapter 1 in *Unblemished!*

Rodrigo, Joseph. Quoted in Shirley's Wellness Café.com (2005)

Schulze, Richard. healing-source.com

Shea, Sheila. "What is Colon Hydrotherapy?" shea.com

"Side Effects," *The PDR Family Guide to Prescriptions*. naturalessentials.com/accutane.htm

Simmons (no first name given), quoted in tuberose.com
    skinandhealth.com

"Social Impact of Acne," *AcneNet.*
    skincarephysicians.com

Sodhi, Virender. "Ayuredic Science Update."
    ayuredicscience.com

Sultzberger and Zaldens (first names not given), quoted in
    "The Social Impact of Acne." (1948).

"Take Control Now!" Chapter 1 in *Overcoming Your
    Objections* (na).

Thoreau, Henry David. Quoted in "An Apple a Day."
    vegparadise.com

T Nguyen2, "Drug-Resistance Web Presentation."
    fubuni.swarthmore.edu

Toxicology-Info.com

Tsao, Amy. "The Changing Face of Skin Care," *Business
    Week Online* (December 2004).

tuberose.com

Volk, Tom. "Tom Volk's Fungus of the Month for
    January 1999." TomvolkFungi.net

wholehealthmd.com

Work, Fredrick, quoted in *JET*.